A NEW CYCLE

Your Guide to a Better Period, Naturally

A COLLECTION BY GLADRAGS

The information presented in this book is intended for education and empowerment, and is not a substitute for advice, diagnosis, or treatment from a licensed medical professional. This book does not provide medical advice and should not be construed as an attempt to offer or render a medical opinion or otherwise engage in the practice of medicine. The creators of this book shall not be held liable for any direct or indirect damages or injury that result in your use of the content or techniques discussed in this book.

DEDICATION

This guide is dedicated to women everywhere who believe (or have hope) that their cycle is something more powerful than a monthly inconvenience. To every woman who has inspired us with her wisdom, who has helped to break down the social taboos surrounding menstruation, who has made a choice to embrace the power of her body's natural cycle: this book is for you.

CONTENTS

....

INTRODUCTION

Does your period feel like a curse? Do irritability, bloating, cramps, and moodiness leave you wishing for your cycle to just disappear? Are painful periods holding you back from embracing your full feminine self? If so, this book is for you. If you already celebrate your cycle, we challenge you to use this book as a tool to deepen your connection with your body.

In this guide, you'll learn how to improve your menstrual cycle, with help from some of our favorite experts in women's health. From uterine alignment to Ayurveda, you'll be given the tools to take control of your health—naturally.

We encourage you to designate a special notebook to record the pieces that most inspire you as you read. Journaling is a powerful way to deepen your understanding of yourself and bring hidden emotions to the surface. Each chapter concludes with reflection prompts for your journal, as well as an action plan—your next steps to a better cycle. Following these steps will guide you on your path to a happier, healthier period.

As you read, you may encounter old habits to unlearn or negative emotions to transform. We hope you will be patient with yourself on this journey, and listen carefully to the signals your body is sending you.

Your cycle is not a curse. It's an opportunity to take advantage of your unique feminine power and create a more joyful life. Are you ready to meet your flow each month with an open heart? Let's begin. Your new cycle awaits.

CHAPTER 1

···

Fertility Awareness

by Ashley Annis

What do you think of when you hear the word *fertility*? Pregnant bellies and babies? Specialists and tests? Complete confusion? This word often brings up ideas and feelings only associated with pregnancy, but did you know that you can understand, appreciate, and be totally connected to your fertility and your fertility cycle even if you aren't trying to get pregnant?

This chapter will explain how to chart your cycle using the sympto-thermal method of fertility awareness and why it is an amazing practice for women in all different phases of life, including: young women just beginning to menstruate, sexually active women who don't want to conceive, and women who simply want to be more aware of their fantastic feminine bodies. You will begin to understand how the method works by looking at the hormones of the feminine cycle and what those hormones do inside your body during the time between periods. Then we will dive into the two main fertility signs we chart when practicing fertility awareness. And finally, but possibly most importantly, we will discuss the amazing benefits to charting your cycle—knowing what is normal for you, making sense of the different emotions and feelings you go through each cycle, and becoming more confident and connected to your own body.

Let's start with discussing our cycle in detail. Red menstrual blood marks the beginning of a new cycle. The sight and feeling of this blood turns our attention to our wombs (often in a negative way), but the shedding of our uterine lining is not the only thing happening during this time. Snug inside the ovaries are immature eggs, each encased in a little sac called a follicle. During the first phase of the cycle, ten to twelve of these immature eggs are stimulated and begin to grow. We call this part of the menstrual cycle—which includes menstruation and the development of the follicles—the follicular phase. Please note, the follicular phase can vary in length from cycle to cycle and from woman to woman. Things like stress, sickness, and traveling can affect the length of the follicular phase. Some women have long follicular phases, and some have short. These are all normal and healthy. The key hormone of the follicular phase is estrogen. This lovely lady hormone, secreted by the ever-growing follicles, holds many jobs, including stimulating the uterine lining to grow in preparation for a potential pregnancy and activating cervical crypts (small pockets on the inside of the cervix) to secrete cervical fluid. Cervical fluid, which will be discussed later in this chapter, is possibly one of the most amazing benefits to navigating the world in a female body. It may not sound like your favorite topic now, but hang with me—it's amazing!

The Female Fertility Cycle

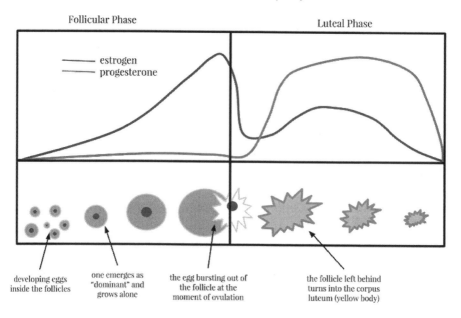

Follicular Phase

Luteal Phase

estrogen
progesterone

developing eggs inside the follicles

one emerges as "dominant" and grows alone

the egg bursting out of the follicle at the moment of ovulation

the follicle left behind turns into the corpus luteum (yellow body)

But back to our cycle: at some point during the follicular phase, one of the ten to twelve developing eggs emerges as dominant (except in the case of fraternal twins or triplets, where two or more eggs continue to grow together). The rest of the follicles are reabsorbed into the body, and the dominant follicle grows alone. Eventually, estrogen production reaches a limit, which triggers the dominant egg to burst through the follicle and the ovarian wall, leaving them both behind. Ovulation has occurred! The egg is swept up by tiny finger-like projections on the ends of the fallopian tubes called fimbria, which direct the egg into one of the tubes after ovulation. The egg can only live for twelve to twenty-four hours, and if it is not fertilized by sperm during that time, it is reabsorbed.

We are now in the luteal phase, the second half of the cycle, which contains quite a bit of action as well. Remember the follicle left behind in the ovary? After ovulation, it goes through an amazing transformation. The follicle turns into the *corpus luteum,* or yellow body, and secretes progesterone, which is the main hormone of the luteal phase. Progesterone, like estrogen, has several important jobs: continuing the development of the uterine lining, keeping the uterine lining from being shed, and preventing the body from ovulating again. Progesterone also raises body temperature, which will come in handy later when we discuss cervical fluid and how to chart your cycle.

The corpus luteum pumps out progesterone for about twelve to sixteen days, which keeps the uterine lining intact. If fertilization and pregnancy occur, the body says to the corpus luteum: "Hey! Keep producing progesterone! We have a baby here, and we don't want that uterine lining to be lost." However, if the message isn't sent, progesterone production ceases, and the uterine lining is shed. A new cycle begins.

Make sense? The whole cycle is geared toward a potential pregnancy. Even though *we* may not be planning on pregnancy every cycle, our body goes through all the preparations as if we were. This may seem strange to those of us who are not ready to have a baby; all those preparations—the uterine lining, the cervical fluid, the progesterone—for

3

nothing? We may not use those subtle signals for pregnancy purposes, but we can use them in other ways: to connect us to our bodies, to grow in our understanding of our cycle, and to appreciate ourselves.

Although it may come as a surprise at first, one of the most empowering parts of having a uterus is the ability to observe and understand your cervical fluid! Cervical fluid, which you may remember is secreted by the cervical crypts, is an alkaline fluid that the female body produces each cycle. This special fluid has three important jobs. First, it decreases the acidity of the vaginal environment. Second, it acts as a medium in which sperm can swim to meet the egg. Finally, it gives women information about where they are in their cycle. As menses comes to an end, the building estrogen in the body stimulates the crypts to produce more and more cervical fluid. As estrogen builds, women experience a progression of fluid called the "fertile wave." During the fertile wave, the fluid will generally start off a bit tacky, pasty, white, or dry. Within a few days, it will move toward a wetter-quality fluid, looking sort of creamy or lotiony, and eventually turn into peak-type fluid, which is super stretchy and looks a lot like raw egg white. This peak-type fluid is the most fertile type of fluid (which means it is the best type of fluid for sperm) and is secreted right before ovulation occurs. Of course, this is just an example of what a fertile wave could look like. Different women have different variations of normal.

It makes sense if you think about it: our bodies are programmed to reproduce, and the better chance the sperm has to survive, the better chance a woman will get pregnant. Right before a fully matured egg is available, the body produces a fluid that will assist the sperm as much as possible. After ovulation occurs, the fluid is no longer needed—reproductively speaking—so the body stops producing it. When tracking your cervical fluid, the following pattern can often be seen: bleeding, maybe some days with no fluid, first sign of fluid (tacky, sticky, dry), building fertile wave, peak-day fluid (wet and slippery, like egg whites), and then back to a tacky fluid or a dry luteal phase. This cycle of fluid can be recorded on a fertility awareness chart. It can give a woman a clear idea of when she is about to ovulate and confirm once ovulation happens—she will see fertile fluid and will know ovulation is close, and then she will see her fluid drying up and know that ovulation has occurred.

The second part of charting your cycle is BBT, or basal body temperature, which is just a fancy term for your temperature when you wake up first thing in the morning. At night while you sleep, your body is resting and resetting for the next day. When you take your temperature first thing in the morning, you are taking your temperature with a blank slate; you haven't been moving around, eating, thinking, or talking, and all those things can change your body temperature ever so slightly. Why does BBT matter for fertility awareness? If you remember from our hormone lesson, after ovulation the follicle turns into the corpus luteum and begins producing the hormone progesterone, which is a heating hormone. When there is progesterone in your system, it will raise your body temperature a noticeable amount. If you are taking your temperature consistently, and you know what your body temperature range is before ovulation occurs, you will know you've ovulated because you will see your temperature rise.

The last part of practicing fertility awareness is recording your cervical fluid and BBT observations on a chart. Fertility awareness charts will include a space for recording cervical fluid, a range of numbers for each day so you can record your temperature, the cycle day, the day of the week, and space for any additional information you want to add. Some women use phone apps, while others use paper charts. Both ways of charting have pros and cons, and if you choose to practice fertility awareness you should use a chart that feels right and will help make your practice sustainable.

Practicing fertility awareness may seem like a lot of work, and at first, it sort of is! Not only do you have to make the practice a habit (your chart won't give you much information if you don't actually record your observations every day), but there are also strong cultural barriers you may have to fight against. It's not always considered normal to check your cervical fluid every day or to think so much about your reproductive system. You may be wondering, is it really worth it? What will this practice teach me? What will I gain? For women who are sexually active, the practice provides a way to prevent pregnancy without the use of hormones. This freedom—not needing hormonal birth control—is enough motivation to learn the method for some women, but even those who aren't dealing with birth control issues can find many reasons why practicing fertility awareness is amazing. These reasons include: the education and experience to make informed decisions about your health and wellness, a way to check in with and be connected to your body and the earth, and greater confidence in yourself.

How do you feel when you see your doctor or OB-GYN? Is it a gentle, positive experience, or do you feel pressure to make choices you don't want to make? For many women, it is frustrating when someone they barely know understands their body better than they do, but this doesn't have to be the case. Charting your cycle gives you the freedom to make informed, comfortable decisions about your reproductive health rather than being forced into a choice you don't want to make. Through the practice of charting, you will learn what is normal for you, which balances out the conversations you have with your doctor. Normally when going to see the doctor, the patient simply tells the doctor what is wrong, and the doctor tells the patient what to do. When a woman charts her cycle and knows her body, she can not only tell her doctor what she thinks is wrong, but also share what she knows from experience about her body. Your doctor has years of practice and experience with diseases and sickness, and you can have cycles and cycles of experience with your unique, special body. Not every woman has a "textbook" body and cycle, so understanding the ins and outs of your own cycle can allow you to work *with* your doctor.

You can also use your fertility awareness chart to record other health and wellness issues, including food allergies or sensitivities, sickness and pain, emotional ups and downs, relationship difficulties, energy levels, and much more. When you write down your observations, you become more aware of what you eat, the way you feel, and how you treat yourself.

Checking in with all of the different parts of your overall wellness—physical, mental, emotional, and even spiritual—can help you to take better care of yourself, which is always a good thing to do. Taking a moment to fill out your chart every day can also become a little ritual. So often, women are focused on taking care of others and don't give enough care to themselves. Even if you spend just three minutes a day thinking about your cervical fluid and writing down your emotions, you are forming the habit of giving time to yourself. Learning self-care is an important piece of overall health and wellness, and practicing fertility awareness can get you moving in the right direction.

As you pay closer attention to your body and your cycle, you may notice different patterns that emerge. Not only will you know where you are in your cycle (ie: "I will probably ovulate in a couple days!" or, "I am about halfway through my luteal phase and will start bleeding in about seven days."), but you might also notice different feelings, emotions, and energy at different points in your cycle. For instance, some women have more creative and social energy around the time of ovulation, so they plan creative projects, make new connections, and work hard to accomplish their goals during this time. Some experience a desire to be still, quiet, and calm during menstruation, and tend to be more introverted and reflective while they are bleeding. However, these are just examples, and there is no right or wrong way to feel. The important thing is to recognize the different ways you feel and perceive your life during the different phases of your cycle. You can use the natural ebb and flow of your energy to make sure you get all the things you need: time to be super social, time to draw inward and reflect, time to work and create, and time to rest and relax. The female body is amazing since it gives us a built-in schedule for all the things we need to feel happy and whole.

Can you see how fertility awareness is all about empowerment, connection to your body, and understanding your uniqueness? The practice teaches you the language your body speaks (your cervical fluid and BBT patterns), and gives you a way to enter in the conversation when you write it all down on a chart. Often we are taught to hide our natural selves—especially menstruation since it can be seen as "dirty" or "weird"—but through the practice of fertility awareness, we begin to normalize our beautiful cycle, which helps us to feel proud and excited to be women. This knowledge and pride translates to confidence about our identity, our feelings and ideas, and the way we move through the world. Let your cyclical nature be your foundation, your constant, your secret, and your power. Your time to bleed at the beginning of each cycle is a fresh start: let yourself bleed and let go. Your fertility is a gift: create and love! Your cycle is a helper, not a hindrance. Love your body, but most importantly, love yourself!

Reflection Prompts

Many women ignore the nuances of their cycle until they try to become pregnant. Consider your own current awareness of your fertility and how it has changed over time as you answer the questions below in your journal.

What is your current relationship with your own fertility and menstrual cycle? What would you like that relationship to be like in one year?

Write down three ways you can become more aware of your body and its natural rhythms this month.

Write down and reflect on any strong reactions or emotions that came up during this chapter.

Your Next Steps Toward a Better Cycle

Read:

- *Taking Charge of Your Fertility* by Toni Weschler

- *The Garden of Fertility* by Katie Singer

- *Her Blood is Gold* by Lara Owen

Chart:

- Use the chart on the following page or download and print your own fertility awareness chart at www.lovelyfertility.com

- Make a habit of charting daily!

Learn more:

- Sign up for an online fertility awareness class series at www. lovelyfertility.com

Ask questions:

- Have questions? E-mail Ashley at lovely.fertility.class@gmail.com

Empower:

- See the beauty of your body. Love yourself!

name _____ chart # _____ month _____ year _____

longest cycle _____ shortest cycle _____ this cycle _____ luteal phase _____

Symbol	Description
* menses	heavy bleeding
(*) spotting	
— dry	any cervical fluid present
CF	peak cervical fluid
(CF) peak cervical fluid	
❋ peak day	
LM luteal mucus	
I infertile BIP	

description (ie: heavy bleeding, stretchy/ wet fluid in the AM. reading obscured by semen or spermicide, cloudy fluid all day, etc.)

additional information (i.e. stress, pain, PMS, nutrition, vaginal sensation etc.)

♡ intercourse with barrier method	
♥ unprotected intercourse	
W withdrawal	
O no genital to genital contact	
• firm/ closed cervix	
O in between cervix	
O soft/ open cervix	

cycle day / date / temperature time / symbol / temperature / cervix / intercourse/ method / birth control p + 4 / t 3

Honey-Grilled Figs with Coconut Cream

by Nicole Jardim

You'll fall in love with this luscious dessert! In many cultures, figs are considered an aphrodisiac and symbol of fertility. When split in two, they resemble the female reproductive organs and when left whole, the male reproductive organs.

Honey-Grilled Figs

4 figs, halved lengthwise

3 T Honey

1 T natural almonds, chopped finely (optional)

Set the oven to broil. Line a baking tray with aluminium foil. Place the figs, cut side up, on the baking tray. Drizzle the figs with honey. Cook for five to six minutes until figs are soft and golden. Divide the figs and add a dollop of coconut cream to each. Sprinkle with the almonds.

Coconut Cream

1 can full-fat coconut milk (refrigerated overnight)

1-2 tsp powdered xylitol

½ tsp pure vanilla extract

Scoop the top layer of white, fatty coconut milk into a medium mixing bowl (discard the coconut water or save it for smoothies). Blend the chunks of coconut milk with a hand mixer on high speed for fifteen to twenty seconds, just until the mixture turns to liquid. Add the xylitol to taste and mix until combined. Add the vanilla extract and blend on high speed for one to two minutes, until light and creamy.

Introduction to Lunar Charting

. . . .

Connecting more deeply with nature and your cycle through alignment with the moon

by Emily Ruff

Cycles of all kinds drive our biological functions and give rhythm to our life. From seasonal cycles to our daily sleep cycles, to our heartbeats and our breath, we are constantly immersed in layers upon layers of rhythm.

These rhythms, both within and outside our body, make up the symphony of our life. When those rhythms are in harmony, we feel in sync with our surroundings. When those rhythms are out of balance, we may feel the dissonance in our emotions, our energy, or our focus.

As women, one of the notable external cycles that influences our internal rhythms is the cycle of the moon. The lunar cycle follows a 29.5-day pattern, where the amount of light reflecting toward the earth shifts from "new" (or dark moon) to "full" (or bright moon).

This cycle has been long known by our ancestors—and recently reaffirmed by modern science—to have a physical, emotional, and biological effect on the human body. The shifts in the moon's relationship to the earth—in the areas of light and gravity, most notably—affect our endocrine system and nervous system in marked ways that adjust our sleep, energy, mood, and hormone regulation. In our modern times, we document more emergencies, more chaotic energy, and more accidents during the full moon. We document an increase in childbirth, too. Our gardens are also influenced by the energy of this cycle, and the phases of the moon offer a backbone to the planting advice found in such classics as the *Farmers' Almanac*.

Because our menstrual cycle follows a turning that is similar in length to the turning of the moon's phases, the menstrual cycle has long been connected in many traditions to the cycle of the moon. Not only does our menstrual cycle follow a rhythm of roughly twenty-eight days like the moon's cycle, but it is also highlighted by two key events—ovulation and menstruation—at points similar to the highlight of the moon's cycle: new moon and full moon.

In current times, creating an intentional practice of connecting with the moon's cycle is more important than ever. Our ancestors once felt the shifts in lunar energies in a very apparent way, through the strikingly visual fluctuation between its light as it waxed and waned from new to full and back to new again. These days, the trappings of the modern world muffle the moon's influence over us. For instance, if you live in an urban area, you may have a constant full moon outside your window every night of the month thanks to streetlights. Thus, reconnecting with the powerful ebb and flow of the moon's energy becomes a practice we must take on with mindfulness.

Realigning with this practice can be as simple as tracking your monthly cycle on a moon calendar. Through brief but frequent connection with a personalized lunar chart, you can begin to attune your inner cycle to the influence of the moon's energy. As you become familiar with how your internal cycle dances with the cycle of the moon each month (maybe you menstruate at the new moon and ovulate at the full moon, or the reverse, or you swim a bit between the two), you follow the energy patterns of nature in more awareness of the beauty in this relationship. You develop a deeper understanding of and connection with your body, the earth, and the cosmos. This connection gives us many gifts, including feeling grounded and supported, a stronger sense of intuition, and access to our body's wisdom.

For those of you new to a relationship with the moon's cycle, my first recommendation is to keep a moon calendar with your personal menstrual cycle charted within it. This can be done by adding the lunar endpoints of new and full moon to your current daybook, purchasing a calendar that integrates lunar cycles into regular date keeping (We'Moon is a favorite of mine), or posting a dedicated lunar calendar on your wall and adding small notes to it. I keep a basic moon calendar posted next to my bathroom mirror. Each day, I get to wake up and check in with the position of the moon's cycle. This keeps me connected daily to the energy of the lunar relationship.

I also make note on my moon calendar of when my own moon—my menses—joins me, so I can compare over the seasons how my cycle relates to the moon's cycle. For many of my female clients who have what they would term an irregular cycle (one that comes at variable dates and lengths each month) many find that just by tracking their menstrual cycle on a moon calendar over a season, the awareness of these rhythms brings their own body's cycle into a schedule that is more predictable within the moon's rhythm.

How our own cycle creates harmony with the moon's cycle can be a teaching, too. Some suggest that if our menses falls on a new moon and our ovulation on a full moon, our cycle is aligned with the fertility of the earth and her sister moon. When we bleed, we tend to go within ourselves—an energy supported by the dark moon—and when we ovulate, we tend to seek more social connection—an energy supported by the bright full moon. Many times, this alignment is referred to as the White Moon Cycle.

Others offer the idea that if our menses falls with a full moon—sometimes referred to as the Red Moon Cycle—that is symbolic of our nurturing energies offered out to our community, our peer group, and those surrounding us. Of course, still others among us may menstruate on the first quarter, last quarter, or somewhere in between. All these harmonies can be healthy and connected. The simple act of conscious awareness provides a tool that nourishes our relationship and deepens our insight.

After working with hundreds of women to chart their menstrual cycles alongside a lunar cycle, my sense is that where our personal cycles fall in harmony with the lunar cycle gives us a window of understanding into our unique and intimate relationship with the energies of nature. Whether we bleed with the new moon, full moon, or neither, through keeping a lunar/menses chart, we can tap into an alignment of energy that comes with deepening our connection with the moon's cycle. Over time, patterns will emerge that can provide meaningful insight into our personal health, our emotional process, and our connection to the universe.

Reflection Prompts

In this modern age of smartphones and constant connection, finding time and space to interact with nature can be difficult. As you journal, you are encouraged to take time to be present with nature—whether you sit outside under a tree or simply place fresh flowers in your bedroom.

Do you take note of the moon's cycles? What natural cycles do you find meaningful?

Spend a few minutes detailing the activities you enjoy that enhance your connection to the earth. If you feel disconnected from nature, brainstorm ways to deepen your awareness of the natural world.

Write down and reflect on any strong reactions or emotions that came up during this section.

CHAPTER 2

....

Align Thy Uteri

by Barbara Loomis

Proper alignment of the uterus ensures optimal flow of blood, lymph, energy, and nerve conduction. Without proper flow, pain, hormonal imbalance, and dysfunction will result. Years ago I had a uterus that was flexed forward (anteflexed), and my periods were very painful. My poor little uterus had to twist and turn each month to move the blood that was trapped at the fundus (the opposite end from the cervix). Imagine if you were permanently flexed at the waist with your head level with your knees. Even if you were able to maintain this position, your arterial, venous, and lymph systems would be impaired. Let's face it: you weren't designed to be flexed forward all the time, and neither was your uterus.

> *"When the uterine muscle lacks proper oxygen, acid builds up, and cramping is the result. Acid accumulation and lack of oxygen cause an inability to flush menstrual fluids properly and completely, resulting in an accumulation of these fluids on the uterine membrane. The accumulated fluids are referred to as "induration," hardened and dry. Pain worsens each cycle as the uterus has more indurated, thick blood to expel while working against acid accumulation, poor oxygen, and malposition."* **Dr Rosita Arvigo, Naprapathic physician**

Where the heck is my uterus?

The uterus sits between the bladder and rectum, ideally with a little space in between the organs. If the uterus is not in proper position it can affect the function of the surrounding organs and the uterus itself. Consider this: the uterus weighs about four ounces when you're not menstruating, and can double in size (to eight to ten ounces) right before and during your period! That's a lot of extra weight on your rectum or bladder, depending on which way your uterus is tipped. The uterus can also be leaning to the left or the right, causing an array of other problems.

But my doctor said it was normal to have a tipped uterus!

It may be common, but it's not natural to have your uterus hugging your rectum or squashing your bladder. I'm always surprised to hear women say that their OB-GYN told them that a tipped uterus doesn't cause problems. When looking at the images above, it's obvious to me how a shifted uterus can interfere with normal functioning of the surrounding organs.

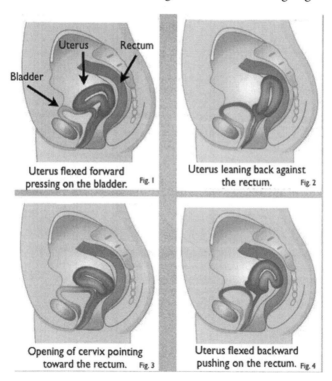

Uterus flexed forward pressing on the bladder. Fig. 1

Uterus leaning back against the rectum. Fig. 2

Opening of cervix pointing toward the rectum. Fig. 3

Uterus flexed backward pushing on the rectum. Fig. 4

Even the book *Obstetrics and Gynecology*—the very textbook these skeptical physicians and nurses used in medical school—indicates that a retroflexed (figure 4) and retroverted (figure 2) uterus is associated with dyspareunia (painful intercourse) and dysmenorrhea (painful periods).[1] I also found that my anteflexed (figure 1) uterus limited my bladder's capacity to hold urine.

> *"The bladder and the uterus are highly interdependent... Normal urogenital functioning is impossible if the uterus is anteverted and anteflexed, or if its fasciae are restricted."* Jean-Pierre Barral, osteopathic physician[2]

How do I know if I have a wandering womb?

Your doctor may tell you, or you may have to ask during a pelvic exam if you have a tipped uterus. Although there can be dietary, environmental, or other causes for the following symptoms, a shifted uterus can be a contributing factor if not the main cause. This list of symptoms includes painful or irregular menses; amenorrhea, or no menstruation at all; headaches or dizziness with menses; varicose veins; fertility challenges or difficult pregnancy or delivery; endometriosis or endometritis; uterine polyps; painful intercourse; PMS; uterine infections; frequent urination; ovarian cysts; vaginitis; and difficult menopause. *Wow*, right?

The following pelvic alignment and self-massage suggestions are beneficial to anyone with a pelvis—male or female, posthysterectomy, postmenopausal, tipped uterus or perfectly aligned uterus. These techniques help to optimize flow of the major systems of the body. Who doesn't need that?

Blood carries hormonal messages and feeds every cell of the body with oxygen and nutrients. The lymph system is like the police force and garbage collector; when they both go on strike pathological debris builds up, and mayhem ensues.

But wait. Was I born like this?

Probably not. Common causes of a displaced uterus include wearing high-heeled shoes, falls on the sacrum (the lowest part of the spine above the tailbone), chronic straining during bowel movements, difficult birthing experiences, motor vehicle accidents, surgical procedures, and poor pelvic alignment.

Let's talk pelvic alignment.

Your uterus is attached to the inside of your pelvis, so if your pelvis is out of alignment, your uterus will be out of alignment as well. For instance, if the pelvis is posteriorly tilted (think tucked tailbone), the uterus may be pushed back against the rectum or down toward the vaginal opening (prolapse). An aligned pelvis is when the anterior superior iliac spine (the uppermost part of the front of the pelvis) and pubic symphysis (locate it by moving your hand down your soft belly until you feel a bone) are in vertical alignment while standing or sitting.

Sounds technical, right? It is, yet it's also a very simple concept, one that's important to understand. Now that you know what an aligned pelvis is, you don't want to force your body into that position by tightening against muscles that have been restricted from years of sitting in chairs. You will need to lengthen the muscles that are pulling your skeleton out of alignment first. This may take time; be patient and gentle with your body.

How do you do this? Ideally, you should see a Restorative Exercise™ Specialist to have your alignment assessed and learn specific exercises that restore your muscles to the correct length. There are some simple things you can start doing today to help influence your alignment:

- **Transition out of positive heeled shoes,** or shoes that elevate your heel higher than the ball of your foot. Elevated heels tilt the pelvis and contribute to pelvic floor dysfunction. You may think those heels make you look sexy, but there's nothing sexy about wearing adult diapers at age forty! I gave all my high-heeled shoes away to people I don't like. (Just kidding...I kept a couple of pairs.) Of course, you can wear a pair of heels once in a while if you absolutely can't find the right flats to go with your special outfit. If you have been wearing positive heeled shoes for most of your life, transition into flats over time to allow your shortened calf muscles to lengthen slowly, carefully, and without undue stress.

- **Get off the couch**. Why not get on the floor while watching a movie? You could stretch for two hours while you are down there. Sitting in a chair all day creates a flat butt, a weak pelvic floor, pelvic congestion, and a cranky uterus.

- **Use bolsters instead of chairs**. One of the great things about using bolsters or getting on the floor is that you get to use your gluteus maximus (butt muscles that give shape to your booty) when you transition to standing or squatting. Strong glutes are not only important for a nice booty, but also essential to maintaining the correct sacral position and a strong pelvic floor.

- **Walk more—and then walk some more**. Walking with an aligned pelvis creates a healthy pelvic floor and a happy uterus.

In short, using your body the way it was designed to be used will help optimize flow within and around the reproductive organs.

Can uterine position be corrected without surgery?

Good news—yes! Sometimes following the above pelvic alignment suggestions is enough to shift uterine position; sometimes you may need a little assistance. Arvigo Techniques of Maya Abdominal Therapy® (ATMAT) is a noninvasive, external massage technique that gently guides the uterus back to its optimal position. Guiding the uterus back to her ideal position is not painful, but is a nurturing and relaxing treatment that improves organ function by releasing congestion from the abdomen and internal organs. ATMAT applies massage, herbology, and Naprapathic-inspired corrections with ancient Mayan healing techniques. Dr. Rosita Arvigo, DN, developed these techniques after apprenticing with Don Elijio Panti, one of the last of the Traditional Maya Shaman of Central America. ATMAT combines modern science with traditional healing and wisdom to produce a holistic path to physical, emotional, and spiritual well-being.

So what actually happens in a session?

Your ATMAT practitioner will massage the area from above your pubic bone to the bottom of your ribcage, as well as your sacrum, hips, mid and low back. Why the back? The ligaments that suspend the ovaries connect all the way up to the third lumbar vertebrae of your low back. If your lower back muscles are tight they can interfere with blood flow to and from the ovaries.

Your ATMAT practitioner can teach you a specific massage for uterine alignment, but in the meantime you can start massaging your own belly to soften the abdominal layers, improve blood flow, and connect you with your internal messages so you become more body-aware for overall health.

First, there are actually times when you should *not* perform lower belly massage. Those times are when you:

- may be pregnant.

- are menstruating or are five days before your period.

- are using an IUD.

- have an active infection or certain cancers (get permission from your doctor).

- are recovering from surgery (usually six to eight weeks depending on physician approval).

- have an inguinal hernia. Always use caution with hernia repair, and seek professional guidance.

If none of these apply, you might want to try this nurturing belly massage on yourself. Ready?

Breathe in, expanding your rib cage. Take several deep breaths until you feel present in your body.

Starting at your navel, use the pads of your index and middle fingers to gently massage in tiny spiral motions. Take your time working through the tension around your navel. Breathe into tight areas to massage it from the inside.

Keep the spirals tiny, but expand out in a larger clockwise spiral until you cover your entire abdomen. Listen to your body—sometimes it feels good to massage more deeply, and sometimes your body will respond better to a lighter touch. Experiment with what works best for you. Don't force anything. Work with your body.

After you massage your entire abdomen with the little spirals technique, knead your belly with the heels of your hands, back and forth like cat paws from side to side.

Rest with one hand on your uterus and one hand on your heart. Feel the loving warmth radiate from your hands as you smile into your heart. Smile down gratitude, kindness, and compassion. Let your smiling energy warm and soften your jaw, neck, chest, upper back, and heart. If you have trouble smiling into your heart, call in all the loving energy from those who have ever loved or cared for you—friends, family, pets, spirit guides, or angels—those who feel safe. Let the vibration of love fill and soften your heart, flow over into your chest and into your pelvis, connecting your heart with your uterine energy. Let this loving energy flow through your fallopian tubes, around your ovaries, and in and around your uterus. Do this for as long as feels comfortable.

Now place your thumb tips together at your navel. Your index fingers should meet in a V formation. Your ovaries should be just beneath the layers of abdominal tissues that lie beneath your pinkies. Tune into your ovaries. Place your palms over your ovaries. How do they feel? Does the left feel different than the right? Do they feel soft, hard, fluffy, warm, or cold? Scan your ovaries and uterus with your mind's eye. How do they look? Is there a color or shape that you see? Don't judge what comes up—just be present and allow the energy to transform as needed. You don't have to figure anything out, only listen as you would listen to a good friend. Where your attention goes, your energy flows. Your body knows what it needs; you just need to learn to listen to its messages. Take your thinking mind out of it.

When you feel finished, give thanks to your body for working hard for you and write down any insights you may have had.

Vaginal steams

A great accompaniment to the abdominal massage is—brace yourself—herbal vaginal steams. Yes, you read that right. Vaginal steams, or *bajos* as they are known in Spanish or *chai-yok* in Korean, have been used for centuries to treat many conditions including painful or irregular periods, endometriosis, infertility, fibroids, cysts, cervical stenosis (narrowing of the cervix), vaginal dryness, and hemorrhoids. For dysmenorrhea, or painful periods, you can do the steams up to three times the week prior to your period or on the first day of your period if you are spotting.

Because of the abundance of blood vessels and mucus membranes, the true essence of oils found in herbs can be more easily absorbed through the walls of the vagina. Vaginal steams also work as a uterine lavage to cleanse the uterine wall of accumulated debris and to nourish the womb on a physical and energetic level. Ready to try it? Read on!

Vaginal steam instructions

Never use a vaginal steam when you are pregnant or think you might be, if you are using an IUD, or if you have an active infection. Avoid steams during herpes outbreaks, since herpes is considered a damp-heat condition and a steam may aggravate the condition. Always consult your doctor if you think you may have a medical condition.

- Collect organic plants with prayer and intention or use dried herbs (use one quart fresh or one cup dried). Some commonly used herbs are basil, calendula, lemon balm, oregano, and rosemary.

  Crush herbs into a large pot with a gallon of water as you give thanks and infuse them with your loving intentions.

  Bring the mixture to a soft boil for five minutes, then steep for ten minutes with the lid on.

  Place the pot under the chair you will use to steam. You may use a wooden chair specifically designed for the purpose, or a U-shaped shower chair. Visit the vaginal steam article on my blog to learn how to easily do your steam on the toilet as well.

  Test the steam on your wrist before sitting down. The membranes of your vagina are sensitive, so you don't want it to feel too hot. Get undressed from the waist down (keep your warm socks on) and sit on the chair with a blanket wrapped around you to keep the steam in the area.

  Sit comfortably for at least twenty minutes. You may choose to meditate, read a book, watch Oprah, or whatever is enjoyable to you (unless it's a Bruce Willis film—some things just don't mix). The heat should feel pleasant. I usually feel the warmth fill my belly and rise all the way up to my heart. If it feels too warm, remove the pot to let it cool a bit.

Rest afterward, stay warm, and do something nurturing for yourself like drinking a warm, herbal tea of raspberry leaf, nettles, and oat straw, or taking a warm bath.

Doing vaginal steams in conjunction with abdominal massage and correcting your pelvic alignment will do wonders for your overall health.

There you have it: several simple yet effective self-care tools you can use to enhance your reproductive health. If you experience painful or irregular cycles, please don't be angry with your uterus. Sometimes pain is a healthy response to an unhealthy situation. Your womb is working hard to maintain homeostasis (balance within) but because of modern life, environmental toxins, diet, and shifted organs, your uterus has to work extra hard to maintain balance. Here's the good news: you now have the tools to remove the obstacles that make your period a dreaded event instead of the sacred and special time it truly is.

Reflection Prompts

There are few body parts more openly complained about by women than the uterus! Choosing to release negativity toward your body is an important step in your journey toward greater health. As you journal, allow your emotions to flow freely without judgment—you can examine your feelings later, after you have transferred them to the page. You may even choose to draw, paint, or express yourself in another creative way.

Write down your feelings toward your uterus and reproductive organs. Reflect on the many embedded emotions you may have toward this powerful area of your body.

Write down and reflect on any strong reactions or emotions that came up during this chapter.

Your Next Steps Toward a Better Cycle

- Do belly massage and uterine meditation every day for at least ten minutes (except for those times that are contraindicated).

- Get an Arvigo Techniques of Maya Abdominal Therapy™ treatment. Find a practitioner near you at www.arvigotherapy.com.

- Walk more. Set a goal of walking at least five miles a day.

- Do the five Restorative Exercises™ on the *"Down There" for Women* DVD, available on www.nurturance.net, or see a Restorative Exercise™ Specialist in your area for a personalized alignment evaluation. If there isn't one in your area, I can help you via Skype sessions, or you can find free alignment information on my blog at http://alignmentmonkey.nurturance.net.

- Do a vaginal steam at least once a month right before your period (see contraindications).

- Sit less—get rid of your couch, lie on the floor to watch movies, get a standing workstation.

- Ditch the high heels!

- Listen to your body.

- Have appreciation for how hard your body is working for you.

1. Barral, Jean-Pierre, *Urogenital Manipulation*, 57.

2. *Obstetrics and Gynecology*, ISBN-10: 0781788072, ISBN-13: 978-0781788076, 6th ed., 37.

CHAPTER 3

....

Your Vagina: An Owner's Guide

How to Keep Your Vagina Healthy, or How to Properly Tend Your Vagina Garden

by Miriam Rosenberg, CNM

The vagina: your lady flower, your hooha, your va-jay-jay. Call it what you will, it is a lovely and complex part of your body. Every vagina is different, and women frequently worry that theirs is somehow "not normal." This chapter is designed to explain the wide variety of normal vaginas and how to properly care for yours. But first, a quick anatomy lesson.

What we commonly think of as the vagina is really an interconnected set of body parts. There's the vulva, which is the external part including the mons (the fatty pad of tissue over the pubic bone), the outer lips (the labia majora), and the inner lips (the labia minora). At the point where the inner lips join at the top is the clitoris, that most lovely and sensitive spot. Fun fact: the part of the clitoris you can feel and see from the outside is actually just the tip of a larger organ that extends deep inside your body! Then there's the vagina itself, which is the flexible corridor that leads to your cervix, the opening of your uterus. The vagina can expand and stretch to accommodate a penis, a baby, fingers, sex toys, spare change, etc. It is not the rigid tube most anatomy textbooks make it out to be.

The inside of your vagina is a moist, warm, acidic environment that is the happy home to a whole host of bacteria, or flora. I think of the vagina as a rainforest. Like a rainforest, there are many different organisms growing, and there is a delicate balance of moisture, acidity, and heat that keeps the ecosystem thriving. Most of the time, your body regulates that balance to keep your vagina healthy. It produces discharge that helps to flush out harmful bacteria or debris. It maintains an acidic environment in your vagina that is preferred by a diverse collection of healthy bacteria. Those healthy bacteria, in turn, crowd out any unhealthy bacteria and fungi that may have gotten in. Like supporting a rainforest, taking care of your vagina means both supporting a healthy ecosystem and not introducing any non-native outsiders.

Since your vagina is a part of you, keeping your vagina healthy is in large part keeping YOU healthy. I often tell my clients that there are six basic things they can do to stay healthy:

- Eat a healthy diet: lots of fruits and vegetables, not a lot of sugar and simple carbs.

- Drink plenty of fluids: preferably water instead of sugary drinks or juices.

- Get enough exercise: good for your mood, your bones, your heart. The list goes on!

- Reduce stress in your life: set limits, go for a hike, take time to breathe.

- Get sufficient sleep: essential for giving your body and mind a chance to recharge.

- Quit smoking: easier said than done, but worth the effort.

These simple choices will give your overall health a boost and will help your vagina stay in balance. In addition, there are some specific things you can do to keep your vagina happy and healthy:

- Only use water and your hands to clean your vagina. In general, your vagina cleans itself through normal secretions. Your vagina doesn't need soap to get clean, and it certainly doesn't need to be roughed up with a loofah. In fact, soaps can irritate your vagina and throw your healthy bacteria out of balance. If you absolutely can't stand the idea of not using soap, use an unscented, mild bar soap, just on the outside of your vagina.

- Wipe front to back. The bacteria from your butt don't belong in your vagina. Wiping front to back keeps them from moving that direction.

- Avoid putting anything scented or dyed on, in, or near your vagina. This includes douches, sprays, scented panty liners or tampons, and strong soaps or detergents. These products can irritate your vagina and disrupt the normal delicate balance, allowing fungi and unhealthy bacteria to overgrow.

- Wear cotton undies and skip the panty hose. Synthetic fibers don't breathe well, and keep heat and sweat trapped inside. A sweaty, warm environment is a breeding ground for unhealthy bacteria to overgrow and cause odors and infections.

- Practice safe sex. Sexually transmitted infections can make your vagina and other assorted lady parts very unhappy. By using condoms correctly, getting your partners screened for STIs before initiating sex, and getting tested yourself, you can reduce your risk of picking up one of these infections and avoid the long-term harms these infections can cause.

- Do your Kegels! Pelvic floor strengthening exercises (also known as Kegels) can help increase blood flow to your vagina, prevent and treat urinary incontinence, and improve your sex life (Dumoulin,

2010). You can identify these muscles by using your vaginal muscles to squeeze a vaginal weight, fingers, or penis. Once you've got the hang of it, you can do Kegels anytime without anyone else knowing!

- Give your vagina the love it needs. Pleasure yourself or have someone else pleasure you. Studies have shown that sex (generally) and orgasms (specifically) have numerous health benefits. Arousal and orgasm increase blood flow to your vagina, improving its elasticity, lubrication, sensation, and ability to fight off infections.

Frequently Asked Questions

What does a healthy vagina/vulva look like?

That's kind of like asking, "What does a healthy nose look like?" Like women, vaginas come in a variety of shapes, sizes, colors, and styles. Some have narrow outer labia, and others have big juicy lips. Some women have tiny inner labia you can't see from the outside. Some have very long inner labia that protrude like flower petals from within the outer labia. On average, inner labia are about three-quarters of an inch long to over two inches long at the longest point. But just like the penis, vaginal tissues can change in size when they're turned on. Arousal brings a tidal wave of blood flow to the area, increasing sensitivity and size. Labial colors can range from black to brown, peachy to pink, purplish-violet to blue! Many women will have some combination of these colors. In addition to being nice window dressing, the vulva serves some pretty useful functions: it acts as a protective screen, keeping unhealthy foreign bacteria out. It also increases friction and lubrication during sex, which for many women increases sexual pleasure.

Many women's sense of what a vagina is supposed to look like comes from some pretty dubious sources: porn, the locker room, and taking care of babies or small children. Many women worry that there's something wrong with their inner labia because they "stick out." Some people feel badly enough about the shape of their vagina that they consider having surgery to "fix" it. This is unfortunate on several levels. First, it shows that many folks think their vagina is shaped wrong, when in reality there is a wide range of normal in terms of vagina shapes. Second, so-called vaginal rejuvenation surgeries can damage the blood and nerve supply. Translation: sex won't feel as good if you get plastic surgery on your vagina. What's the good of having a "perfect-looking" vagina if you can't have as much fun with it?

Which brings me to my next point: what your vagina looks like is less important than what it can DO! Vaginas are pretty amazing: they can bring us sexual pleasure, give sexual pleasure to others, open to bring babies into the world, and give us a sense of connectedness to other women. They are complex and diverse, just like the women to whom they belong. There is an equal degree of diversity among vagina enthusiasts. Some folks find longer, more "flowery" labia to be a huge turn on. Some like a full bush, others prefer trimmed hedges. I invite you to work on loving the unique vagina you were born with and celebrating its unique shape, size, color, and scent.

What should a healthy vagina smell like?

A healthy vagina should smell exactly like a vagina. Just like a good bar of chocolate should smell like...well, chocolate. And the "vagina smell" can be pretty different from lady to lady. Your signature aroma is based on your personal rainforest of bacteria, what you ate for dinner, what type of undies you wear, how and how often you bathe, where you are in your menstrual cycle, and what your glands contribute to the equation. Vaginas are supposed to have a smell; they are a reservoir of scents that help us to attract a mate. An informal poll of folks who have spent a fair amount of time around healthy vaginas yielded the following descriptors: musky, metallic (especially right before a period), pungent, tangy, salty, sweaty, primal, like the ocean, like wet sand, and like "an oyster with a drop of soy sauce on it." Vaginas are definitely not supposed to smell like perfume, roses, peaches, or spring rain! Perfumed sprays and douches are designed to make vaginas not smell like vaginas. Would you want eat a chocolate bar that smelled like Irish Spring?

Sometimes the vagina can get a funky smell reminiscent of fish, garbage, bread, or bleach. This is often because the normal vaginal balance has gotten out of whack: there's something in there that usually isn't. This can be due to a bacterial or fungal infection, the presence of semen after sex, or a sexually transmitted infection. A common response to a funky-smelling vagina is to use a perfumed spray, soap, or douche to cover up the odor. This is problematic in several ways. First, vaginal deodorants don't get rid of the smell, they just add another smell on top. Second, these products can worsen the imbalances that caused the odor in the first place by killing off the healthy bacteria that keep outside invaders in check. Finally, they will not address any underlying problems that are making your vagina smell funky.

To reduce the likelihood of "bad" vaginal odors, see the previous section on how to care for your healthy vagina. If your vagina smells less like a vagina and more like something gnarly, get it checked out by your health care provider. They can do tests for infection, suggest treatments if needed, or even just reassure you that everything is just as it should be.

Should I shave my pubic hair?

Some ladies prefer more hair, some ladies prefer less hair. It depends on what style you like. That said, the hair down there does serve a purpose: it is one of our bodies' methods of keeping out harmful bacteria and other unwelcome guests. It also provides a home for the awesome pheromones that are involved in sexual attraction, so consider that before mowing your lawn. Plus, shaving can cause skin irritation, infections, and rashes (none of which are super sexy), and it takes up valuable time, so some people prefer to just skip it. Waxing and laser hair removal hurt like the dickens, and cost loads of money to boot. If you prefer a less-bushy look, you can always just trim your pubic hair, which gets you the benefits of having some hair down there without the irritation, cost, or pain of other hair removal techniques.

Does discharge mean I have an STD or an infection?

Nope. Your vagina is a self-cleaning oven. That discharge is your body's way of flushing out unhealthy bacteria. Normal discharge can be white, clear, or yellowish. How much vaginal discharge you make varies widely. Normal, healthy women can produce lots of discharge; others are less juicy. As long as you have no itching or odor, and you're reasonable certain you haven't been exposed to any STIs, you're probably just fine. If in doubt, see your friendly, local health care provider.

I keep getting yeast infections! What should I do?

First, make sure it really is a yeast infection. A recent study showed that most women who diagnosed themselves with yeast infections actually had other infections; only 35 percent of women who thought they had yeast actually did (Ferris, 2002). You might protest: "But I've had yeast infections before. I know that's what this is." However, the same study found that women who had previously been diagnosed with yeast infections were no more likely to correctly diagnose themselves than women who hadn't had yeast before. Whoa! Be cautious with self-treating your "yeast infection" that keeps coming back.

If you do have true recurrent yeast infections, I'm sorry. Chronic yeast is tough to live with and tough to treat. Try to eliminate conditions that encourage the growth of yeast: avoid scented panty liners, sprays, and douches, wear breathable cotton underwear without panty hose, and reduce sugar and simple carbohydrates in your diet (especially if you are diabetic; yeast loves sugar). If you are on a high-estrogen birth control pill, consider switching to a lower-estrogen brand.

Unfortunately, there is a lack of scientific evidence supporting the effectiveness of various natural treatments for yeast like garlic, probiotics, tea tree oil, and boric acid suppositories. Then again, there are no pharmaceutical companies making millions selling garlic, so this does not mean these methods are ineffective—only that they have not been well studied. There are studies supporting the efficacy of prescription antifungal pills for treating chronic yeast symptoms and reducing the frequency of infections, but these pills need to be taken on an ongoing basis, and 50 percent of women will start getting recurrent yeast infections again once they stop taking them (Sobel, 2004).

I occasionally recommend that women with tough-to-treat, recurrent yeast try one of the natural treatments for yeast, and I have seen varying degrees of improvement. You can buy probiotic pills, which contain large quantities of healthy bacteria, at most natural food stores. Make sure they are refrigerated, or the bacteria won't survive to do any good. Boric acid suppositories can be purchased at some specialty pharmacies, or you can make your own. In general you can find boric acid powder behind the pharmacy counter (you don't need a prescription). Buy a bottle of that and some size 0 gelatin capsules, available at natural food and supplement stores or online. Open the capsule, use one half to scoop up the powder, pop the other half on, and put it in your vagina before you go to bed at night for prevention of yeast or three times a day for a week for treatment of yeast or bacterial vaginosis. Wearing a panty liner can be a good idea, as some women experience some watery discharge after use. Boric acid is not safe in pregnancy, should never be taken orally, and is not appropriate for everyone, so check with your health care provider before using this treatment.

Reflection Prompts

You may have felt a little uncomfortable while reading this chapter; our societal treatment of women's bodies as primarily sexual objects can make simply reading about healthy vaginas feel embarrassing. Remember that *you* are in control of how you ultimately choose to feel about your own body.

Consider the messages you have received throughout your life about your vagina. Write down these thoughts and where they came from. Do they serve you? What should you keep and what should be let go?

Make a list of what you appreciate about your vagina and vulva.

Write down and reflect on any strong reactions or emotions that came up during this chapter.

Your Next Steps Toward a Better Cycle

- Ditch any fragranced items that you typically use in or around your vagina including douches, sprays, and tampons or panty liners.

- Switch to cotton underwear and avoid panty hose when possible.

- Practice Kegel exercises regularly. First locate the muscles by pretending you are urinating; the muscles you would contract to stop the flow of urine are your PC (Kegel) muscles. To exercise them, simply contract the muscles in an upward motion (you can use a weighted ball inserted in the vagina to help you lift), hold, and relax. Gradually you may increase the weight and the length of the contraction. Make sure to breathe steadily and keep your buttocks, thighs, and abdomen relaxed.

- Grow your appreciation of your vagina through art. Read Eve Ensler's *The Vagina Monologues* and visit The Great Wall of Vagina website at http://www.greatwallofvagina.co.uk/

Dumoulin, C., Hay-Smith, J. (2010) "Pelvic floor muscle training versus no treatment, or inactive control treatments, for urinary incontinence in women," Cochrane Database of Systematic Reviews (1).

Ferris, D.G., Nyirjesy, P., Sobel, J.D., Soper, D., Pavletic, A., Litaker, M.S. (2002) "Over-the-counter antifungal drug misuse associated with patient-diagnosed vulvovaginal candidiasis," Obstet Gynecol 99(3):419.

Sobel, J.D., Wiesenfeld, H.C., Martens, M., Danna, P., Hooton, T.M., Rompalo, A., et al. (2004) "Maintenance fluconazole therapy for recurrent vulvovaginal candidiasis," N Engl J Med 351(9):876.

CHAPTER 4

···

Hormonal Balance for Less PMS

by Dr. Emily Lipinski and Gabriela Delano-Stephens

Before we can discuss hormonal balance, let's clarify a few basics. During the menstrual cycle, your body—or more specifically, your uterus—is preparing for pregnancy. If no egg is implanted in the uterine lining during your cycle, your uterus will shed the lining, you will begin to bleed, and—voilà!—your period begins and the cycle starts over again.

This process is regulated by a number of hormones in the body. So what is a hormone exactly, and how does it have so much power over our body? A hormone, by definition, is a chemical messenger that is released by a gland, a cell, or an organ that will tell cells in other parts of the body what process to carry out. Hormones are like bike messengers taking important information from one part of the body to another. As you can imagine, if your hormones are out of whack, your body will be receiving the wrong messages and making some big mistakes! Therefore it is of utmost importance to maintain healthy, balanced hormones to allow for these messages to be properly sent and received.

The hormones involved in the menstrual cycle are primarily secreted by the ovaries and the pituitary gland, a pea-sized gland at the base of the hypothalamus located in your brain. The menstrual cycle is determined by the number of days from the first day of one's period (the first day of bleeding) to the first day of the next period. A typical cycle is twenty-five to thirty-five days long, with an average woman's cycle spanning twenty-eight days. The menstrual cycle has three phases: follicular, ovulatory, and luteal. The first part of the cycle is the follicular phase, midway through the cycle ovulation occurs (known as the ovulatory phase), and the last part of the cycle is the luteal phase.

The major hormones involved in the menstrual cycle are:

- **Follicle Stimulating Hormone (FSH)**—Released from the pituitary gland in the brain, this hormone stimulates the ovarian follicle to mature. The follicle is a fluid-filled sac containing an egg.

- **Luteinizing Hormone (LH)**—Released from the pituitary gland just before you ovulate, it stimulates the mature follicle to release the egg.

- **Estrogen**—This well-known female hormone shows up mostly in the first part of the cycle. It is produced primarily by the ovaries, but also secreted by the adrenal glands (whose main purpose is to help deal with stress) and adipose tissue (fat tissues). Estrogen helps the uterine lining and the egg develop before ovulation so that both are ready to be fertilized by the sperm and then implanted into the uterine lining.

- **Progesterone**—This is the hormone most abundant in the last part of the cycle because it is produced after ovulation by the corpus luteum (the burst follicle, or egg sac). Progesterone can be produced by other organs in the body, such as the adrenal glands, but to a much lesser degree. Progesterone controls the buildup of the uterine lining and keeps it healthy if pregnancy happens. If there is no pregnancy, progesterone levels fall, and menses begins.

On day one, the day that bleeding begins, estrogen and progesterone levels are low, signaling to the pituitary gland to produce FSH, which encourages the follicle to develop. The mature follicle produces more estrogen, promoting the growth of the uterine lining to prepare for possible pregnancy. As you can see, each hormone "messenger" stimulates the maturation or production of something new.

Around days twelve to fourteen, ovulation occurs, although this can vary from woman to woman, and the exact day of ovulation can also vary slightly from cycle to cycle. Ovulation occurs when the estrogen levels in the body have reached a level high enough to stimulate the release of LH from the pituitary gland, triggering the release of the egg from the follicle. While a female is generally most fertile two days prior to ovulation, there are about six or seven days each month that a woman could become pregnant. This includes the five to six days before ovulation, the day of ovulation, and the day after ovulation.

The ruptured follicle, or corpus luteum, begins to secrete progesterone and estrogen to continue preparing the uterus for pregnancy. If the egg is not fertilized, estrogen and progesterone levels drop around day twenty-eight, and menses begins.

When the hormones involved in menstruation are not in balance, adverse symptoms can arise. Common symptoms of hormonal imbalance are:

- Bloating and water retention

- Acne

- Mood swings

- Fatigue

- Headaches

- Insomnia

- Fibrocystic breasts and breast tenderness

- Sugar cravings

- Dysmenorrhea (menstrual cramping)

- Secondary amenorrhea (you have had your period in the past but are no longer experiencing monthly bleeding)

- Mastalgia (breast tenderness)

These symptoms are common for many women, and are often considered to be an inevitable part of being a woman. However, this is not necessarily true. When a woman's hormones are in balance, she experiences few, if any, PMS symptoms. It is important to note that if you are experiencing the symptoms above, it is always best to seek the care of a health care provider. Some of the symptoms commonly associated with PMS can also be an indication of another underlying disease that should not go undiagnosed.

Given our lifestyle today, it is no surprise that hormonal imbalance and premenstrual syndrome are a standard for many women. Some of the most common reasons for hormonal imbalance are:

Diet—Refined sugar, flour, caffeine, excess alcohol, processed foods, and lack of fiber and nutrients from plant foods can all contribute to hormone imbalance. Additionally, consuming large amounts of red meat, animal fats, and dairy products can increase inflammation in our bodies, worsening symptoms of hormone imbalance and PMS. Not to mention the hormones and antibiotics found in conventional meat and dairy sources: these can also easily add to hormonal disruption.

Stress—Chronic stress can elevate cortisol, a hormone that is associated with experiencing a stressful event. Chronic elevations in cortisol can interfere with the natural balance of hormones in the female body. As many women are aware, stress can also increase the likelihood of making poor diet choices and overindulging in sugar, starches, or fat.

Xenoestrogens—Xenoestrogens are external substances that can interfere with the functioning of the hormonal system, causing unwanted health effects to the organism exposed to the substance and/or the organism's offspring. Common xenoestrogens are man-made chemicals found in fertilizers, pesticides, insecticides, herbicides, cosmetics, and plastics. One simple way to start reducing your exposure is to avoid drinking water out of plastic containers, using glass containers to store your leftovers, and drinking filtered water.

Liver Function—The liver is an important piece of the puzzle when looking at hormonal balance, as this incredible organ breaks down and metabolizes hormones. If the liver is not efficient in processing and metabolizing hormones, hormonal balance is disrupted. Hormonal metabolism in the liver can be slowed due to pesticides, environmental toxins, caffeine, alcohol, sugar, a diet high in low-quality fats, pharmaceutical drugs, or inadequate protein.

Smoking—Smoking can disrupt the balance of female sex hormones (estrogen and progesterone)[1] and may also contribute to obesity. Smoking lowers estrogen levels and affects fertility. Additionally, smoking may lead to earlier onset of menopause.

Sleep—Sleep deprivation decreases leptin, a hormone that regulates appetite. Too little sleep can increase the cravings for fats, sugars, and starches. Sleep is necessary for regeneration and proper functioning of all organs. It is an essential part of any path to wellness.

Tests to Evaluate Hormone Levels

Hormone testing is a great way for you and your health care practitioner to better understand and treat hormonal imbalances causing fertility issues, amenorrhea (lack of period), or mood swings. Symptoms alone may not be enough to properly diagnose a hormone imbalance. For example, a woman's symptoms may indicate an excess of estrogen while in fact she may be low in progesterone. A lowered progesterone level will cause her estrogen to appear high, when in actuality her estrogen levels are fine. In this case, the solution would be to increase her progesterone levels to restore hormonal balance.

Many studies support the use of salivary hormones to understand menstrual cycle profiles. [2-8] Measuring estrogen and progesterone multiple times during a woman's cycle can identify cycle-specific hormonal issues. Bringing your hormones back to balance can be attained through diet, supplementation, and lifestyle adjustments.

Salivary hormone testing can be done with your naturopathic doctor or other health care provider.

Hormone levels can also be measured through urine or blood, however this does not allow for the month-long assessment of hormonal fluctuation. Urine steroid collection involves taking samples over a twenty-four-hour period, while a blood sample is taken once.

Encouraging Healthy Hormones

Diet

A diet to balance hormones must be focused on whole foods and little to no caffeine, refined sugar, and alcohol. Avoid packaged foods and opt for as many fresh fruits and vegetables as possible. It is important to include enough fiber in your diet to keep bowel movements regular. Foods high in fiber include beans, whole grains, nuts, fruits, and vegetables. Two tablespoons of flax or chia seeds added to smoothies, cereal, or salads is a great way to boost fiber intake levels. Blood sugar balance can be encouraged by including protein at breakfast and eating three evenly spaced meals each day. If you are estrogen dominant, foods that contain Indole-3-carbonyl (I3C), such as the brassica family (broccoli, cauliflower, brussels sprouts, kale, and cabbage), can encourage healthy estrogen balance.

Supplements

Supplementation is best when prescribed individually, depending on the cause and specific hormone imbalance. The two listed below are generally well tolerated and well indicated for most hormone imbalances. However, depending on the specific hormone imbalance and cause of imbalance, other remedies may be preferred.

Vitex Agnus Castus (Chastetree Berry) —This herb is well known for its beneficial effects on female hormones and its ability to significantly decrease breast tenderness associated with the menstrual cycle.[9] Numerous studies have also shown reduction in other premenstrual symptoms such as irritability, depressed mood, edema, and headaches. [10-12] Therapeutic effects of vitex have been attributed to its indirect effects on hormones and neurotransmitters, having an overall balancing effect on sex hormones.

Maca —Maca root is widely consumed as a dietary supplement in Peru and is a well-known supplement for improving sexual dysfunction.[13,14] A number of studies suggest that the plant does not contain any estrogens or other phytohormones; rather, maca stimulates the endocrine system to help maintain hormone balance though plant sterols.[15] Therefore, not only does maca seem to improve sexual dysfunction but it is also beneficial to bringing hormones back into balance.

Maca can be taken in powder form mixed into smoothies or sprinkled on top of cereals. Capsules are also available. Maca, like any other hormone-balancing substance, often needs to be consumed for at least three months before beneficial effects may be evaluated or noticed.

There are many other herbs and supplements that can be used to augment hormones. However, because these substances have a specific effect at increasing or decreasing a certain hormone, it is best to seek the advice of a qualified health care professional and have your hormone levels tested to appropriately treat the hormone imbalance.

Yoga

Yoga can be a great way to achieve hormonal balance as it helps to calm the body and reduce stress levels, which ultimately affect hormone balance. Choose yoga classes according to how you feel on a particular day. Go easy on yourself during your period and avoid inversions during menses.

Sleep Hygiene

Sleep is vital for good health and also has a role to play in healthy hormone balance. Many people have trouble sleeping, which can either be attributed to hormonal imbalance or play a role in the imbalance. Listed below are some tips to help you get some quality shut-eye.

Darkness—The hormone melatonin, also known as the darkness hormone, controls the sleep–wake cycles. It is only released when you are in the dark, which is why bright lights before bed could affect the release of melatonin and could interfere with your ability to have restful sleep. Avoiding watching TV or computer screens one hour before bed and dimming the lights in your house an hour or two before you want to go to sleep can help your body prepare for rest. Make sure you are sleeping in a dark room without nightlights or light from outside.

Temperature—Our body temperature drops once we fall into a deep sleep, and overall warm temperatures can interfere with this natural process for good rest. Keeping your room slightly cool or turning the temperature in the house down at night can help you have a better night's rest. Additionally, eating can increase metabolism and body temperature, so it is best to stop eating two hours before bed. If you must, snacking on half an apple or a few nuts can keep hunger at bay until morning.

Noise—It's obvious that noise disrupts sleep. If your sleep is often disrupted due to noises, try using white noise such as a fan or air purifier to block sounds out. Earplugs can also be effective for some.

Reflection Prompts

Take a moment to reflect on how your PMS symptoms are presenting currently and how you will support yourself in balancing your hormones in the future. Pay special attentions to any feelings that may come up for you. Like all health issues, PMS and hormonal balance can be tied deeply to your emotions.

What is your experience with PMS?

Focusing on diet, sleep, and stress, how do you support your menstrual cycle? What habits do you have that are detrimental to your cycle?

Write down and reflect on any strong reactions that came up during this chapter.

Your Next Steps Toward a Better Cycle

· ·

- Eat a diet rich in organic whole foods and fiber, and low in refined sugar, caffeine, and alcohol. Choose organic, hormone- and antibiotic-free meats and dairy.

- Consider having your hormones tested and work with a health care provider that is knowledgeable in balancing hormones naturally and treating premenstrual syndrome.

- Drink eight glasses of water daily, starting your day off with lemon and water to encourage good liver health.

- Consider the herbs vitex agnus castus and maca to balance hormones.

- Use yoga and meditation to help reduce stress levels.

- If you smoke, stop. Seek out a health care practitioner that can assist you in a smoking cessation program.

- Avoid drinking and eating out of anything plastic, and never heat your food in plastics. Choose organic food whenever possible, and limit your exposure to perfumes and other chemicals commonly found in cosmetics that can act as endocrine disruptors. Visit the Skin Deep® Cosmetics Database at www.ewg.org/skindeep for help finding safer products.

1. Mari Pölkki and Markus J. Rantala, "Smoking Affects Womens' Sex Hormone-Regulated Body Form," American Journal of Public Health: August 2009, Vol. 99, No. 8: 1350-1350.

2. Chatterton R., et al, "Characteristics of salivary profiles of estradiol and progesterone in premenopausal woman," J Endocrinol. 2005;186:77-84.

3. Gandara B., et al, "Patterns of Salivary Estradiol and Progesterone Across the Menstrual Cycle," Anna N Y. Acad Sci. 2007;198:446-50.

4. Gann, P., et al, "Saliva as a medium for investigating intra-and interindividual differences in sex hormone levels in premenopausal woman," Cancer Epidemiol Biomark Prev. 2001;10:59-61.

5. Groschl, R., "Current Styus of Salivary Hormone Analysis," 2008;54 (11):1759-69.

6. Ishikawa, M., et al., "The clinical usefulness of salivary progesterone measurement for the evaluation of corpus luteum function," Gynecol Obstet Invest. 2002;53 (1):32-7.

7. Tivis, et al, "Saliva versus serum estradiol: Implications for research studies using postmenopausal woman," Prog Neuropsychopharmacol Biol Psychiatry. 2005;29(5)727-32.

8. Wood, P., "Salivary steroid assays-research or routine?" Ann Clin Biochem. 2009;46:183-96.

9. Carmichael, A.R., "Can vitex agnus castus be used for the treatment of mastalgia? What is the current evidence?" Evid Based Complement Alternat Med. 2008. September 5(3):247-250.

10. Lauritzen, C.H., Reuter, H.D., Repges, R., et al, "Treatment of premenstrual tension syndrome with Vitex agnus castus: Controlled-double blind versus pyridoxine," Phytomedicine 1997;4:183-9.

11. Berger, D., Schaffner, W., Schrader, E., et al, "Efficacy of Vitex agnus castus L. extract Ze 440 in patients with premenstrual syndrome (PMS)" Arch Gynecol Obstet 2000;264:150-3.

12. Prilepskaya, V.N., Ledina, A.V., Tagiyeva, A.V., Revazova, F.S., "Vitex agnus castus: Successful treatment of moderate to severe premenstrual syndrome" Maturitas 2006;55 Suppl 1:S55-63.

13. Brooks, et al, "Beneficial effects of Lepidium meyenii (Maca) on psychological sx and measures of dysfunction in post menopausal woman not related to estrogen or androgen content," menopause 2008 Nov-Dec 15 (6) 1157-62.

14. Shin, et al, "Maca (l. meyenii) for improving sexual dysfunction: a systematic review," BMC complement Altern Med 2010 Aug 6 10:44.

15. Meissner, et al, "Hormone balancing effect of pre gelatinized organic maca (Lepium peruvium chacon) (1) Biochemical and pharmodynamic study on Maca using clinical laboratory model on ovariectomized rats," Int J BioMed Sci 2006 September 2 (3) 260-272.

Sesame Shiitake and Baby Bok Choy

by Nicole Jardim

Bok choy is one of my favorite vegetables because it is super nutrient-dense and very low in calories. Part of the Brassica family, bok choy contains high levels of Indole-3-Carbinol (I3C), a compound that breaks down into Diindolylmethane (DIM). DIM increases estrogen metabolism and helps prevent cancerous changes in your cells, especially breast tissue.

1 small onion, sliced

2 cloves garlic, minced

4 heads baby bok choy, sliced

6 fresh shiitake mushrooms, sliced

1 T toasted sesame oil

1 T gluten-free tamari

1-2 T black sesame seeds

Heat the oil in a frying pan. Add onions and garlic, cooking on medium-low heat for about five minutes. Add the shiitakes, bok choy, and tamari to the pan. Cover and cook for three minutes. Top with sesame seeds and serve.

CHAPTER 5

....

Traditional Chinese Medicine and Your Cycle

by Jessica Kolahi

One of my favorite parts about practicing Chinese medicine is the ability to share insight about the body with my friends, family, and women in my community. I am blown away by the graceful intricacies of our body's systems and natural rhythms. Through my work in my practice, and the words in this chapter, I am on a mission to help women feel empowered to tap into a deeper bodily connection. In this chapter I'll share how ancient Chinese medicine views the menstrual cycle, and gift you with the tools to determine specific imbalances in your own body so you can make purposeful choices and enjoy your menstrual cycle with ease!

Let's start with some of the basics...

The primary goal of Traditional Chinese Medicine (TCM) is to realign the body's innate healing systems. Your body has the power to self-correct and repair. However, modern lifestyles strangle this capacity. As a society, we find ourselves desiring control: control over our environments, control over our bodies, and control over the natural rhythms of the universe. Unfortunately, this desire for control backfires. The more power you try to exert over natural systems, the less you are able to tune in and listen to the powerful messages your body is sharing with you.

TCM recognizes that we are not isolated from nature, and our menstrual cycles are a prime example. For millennia, women have ovulated and bled with the moon, and our lifestyle revolved around these rhythms. We would allow ourselves to rest and reflect during the days of menstruation, when our bodies are more depleted and in need of patience. Then, as we neared ovulation, we would engage in more physical activities and creative endeavors while our energy was naturally at its highest.

Today, however, the menstrual cycle is seen as an inconvenience that women must push through. You can no longer take four or five days off from work to sit and meditate. At times you push against the resistance of your fatigued body, ignoring and quieting the messages it is sending you. This discord with nature causes friction in your body, and over time this friction manifests in physical symptoms.

TCM Theory

According to TCM, the health of the body and the menstrual cycle requires an intricate balance of two substances: qi (pronounced "chee") and blood. Qi can be understood as all of the energy in your body that provides you with the fuel to execute cellular function. On the cellular level, modern theorists equate many functions of qi with those of ATP (adenosine triphosphate). Blood can be described as all the fluid, blood, and lymph in the body. It is responsible for lubricating and nourishing your tissues and organs. Qi can be likened to the intangible "software" of your body that organizes and harmonizes, with blood fulfilling the role of the physical "hardware" in the body.

There are several dysfunctions of qi and blood that can cause negative symptoms in your overall health and menstrual cycle. If there is a deficiency of qi, your body will not have the energy required to generate menstrual blood or mobilize the opening and closing of menses. If there is a deficiency of blood, your body will be unable to spare the fluid and tissue for normal menstruation. Additionally, if the flow of either qi or blood becomes stagnant, you will see signs of increased friction in the body.

Often you will find that your body is suffering from more than one imbalance. This is because no part of your body ever exists in complete isolation of the rest of your body. It is common to find qi and blood stagnation occurring together. Without free-flowing qi, the body lacks the tool to move blood evenly throughout the body. Other times we will find qi and blood deficiency together because the body requires adequate qi as a catalyst in the creation of new blood. It is also quite common to find a combination of deficiency and stagnation in the body.

How can I heal?

To empower you to heal your body and your menstrual cycle, I've created a short quiz to help you determine your personal TCM imbalance. Please note, a TCM self-diagnosis is not a substitution for diagnosis by a licensed acupuncturist or a physician. If you are suffering from a serious medical condition, please seek medical attention by a qualified provider.

As a practitioner, I use acupuncture and herbal medicine to correct these imbalances. However, disciplined self-care is often enough treatment to completely revitalize your body. With greater insight into your body's imbalance, you have the power to heal your menstrual cycle and develop a positive relationship with your moon!

For this quiz, I've divided the menstrual imbalances into four categories: qi deficiency, blood deficiency, qi stagnation, and blood stagnation. Each category has eight diagnostic characteristics for the particular imbalances, which include physical sensations you may experience as well as visual observations that TCM practitioners look for to create diagnoses. To determine your most prevalent imbalance, complete the quiz in regards to your last six menstrual cycles and read the self-care instructions that correlate with your imbalance. If you find you have a tie between more than one imbalance, incorporate suggestions from each category. In Chinese medicine it is possible to have more than one diagnostic syndrome that requires addressing. If you find that you are unsure if you experience any of these symptoms, I challenge you to take time to tune into your body the next time your menses arrives and practice awareness of the signals your body is sending you.

Final food for thought: developing an appropriate self-care regimen is like wildly creative cooking. It takes trial and error to determine the combination of foods and lifestyle choices to create an environment of optimal healing, so be patient with your body while on this journey!

Self Quiz

....

Place a check next to any symptoms you have experienced during your last six menstrual cycles. The section with the most checkmarks indicates your most prevalent imbalance.

Qi Deficiency:

☐ Thin, watery menstruation or blood that is pale pink in color. Light flow, possibly with prolonged spotting

☐ Dull and aching menstrual cramps or cramps that have a feeling of bearing downward on the uterus

☐ Bloating and lethargy

☐ Spotting a few days before menstruation

☐ General fatigue with even lower energy around menstruation

☐ Heavy feeling during menstruation

Blood Deficiency:

☐ Pale-colored blood, which often lasts for only two or three days

☐ Light or scanty bleeding

☐ Minimal pain with menses

☐ Minimal PMS signs

☐ Vaginal dryness and thin endometrial lining

☐ Dizziness, lightheadedness, and poor memory around menses

☐ Lengthy cycles, with delay in arrival of blood flow

Qi Stagnation:

☐ Menses can be thick or dark with clots, or may appear bright red

☐ Flow can be normal, scanty or profuse

☐ Painful cramps that radiate into the genital region

☐ PMS symptoms including irritability, emotionally depressed or easily angered, bloating, breast tenderness, acne that is red or slightly purple

☐ High stress

☐ Delayed ovulation and irregular menstrual cycles, which are variable in length

☐ Difficulty falling asleep at night

Blood Stagnation:

☐ Thick or dark menses with clots

☐ Flow is often profuse at the beginning of the flow and scanty near the end

☐ Severe, stabbing menstrual cramps with tenderness to the touch in the lower abdomenDark-colored acne, lower abdominal distension

☐ Stabbing pain with intercourse

☐ Endometriosis or uterine fibroids, or history of pelvic trauma

☐ Hard masses in the breasts or abdomen

Self-Care Instructions

Qi Deficiency—

When treating qi deficiency, it is equally important to focus on both the generation and conservation of the body's energy reserves.

As a rule of thumb, choose foods that provide easily digestible nutrients, exercise in a manner that is gentle and rejuvenating, and incorporate self-care that builds you up.

Diet

When following a diet to increase qi, choose foods that are packed full of nutrients and easy to digest. Avoid foods that require a large amount of energy to break down and eliminate, as well as foods that increase inflammation in the gut.

Add:

- Complex carbohydrates such as oats, brown rice, and yams

- Steamed and warm vegetables

Avoid:

- Raw vegetables and other uncooked, cold foods

- Dairy products such as milk, cheese, and ice cream

- Sugar and refined carbohydrates

Exercise

Exercise is important for helping your body generate more energy, but it is imperative that you choose exercises that boost, rather than deplete, your qi. Strenuous and exhausting exercises will cause more damage than good if you are very qi deficient. To support your energy, choose activities such as yin yoga, walking, and gentle hikes, and be especially sure to refrain from excessive exercise during menstruation.

Other self-care

Qigong—The ancient practice of the meditative cultivation of qi is called qigong. By deliberately cultivating our qi through this practice, we create a space of regenerative healing in our body, supported by rejuvenating oxygenation of our cells. Qigong courses and instruction can be found locally in most cities or online.

Acupressure—This technique stimulates acupuncture points without the use of needles. It is a form of massage that can be incorporated into a daily routine to promote health and wellness according to your specific TCM diagnosis. According to TCM, our body is covered in acupuncture points that have specific functions of either supporting our qi and blood or moving our qi and blood. To perform acupressure on yourself, hold each point for two to three minutes twice daily with firm pressure. It is normal to feel mild discomfort in these points or in other parts of the body as you activate the deeper energies in your body. Recommended acupressure points for qi deficiency: Stomach 36, Spleen 9, Ren 6.

Food sensitivity testing—One of the most common causes of the lethargy and bloating seen in qi deficiency is ingestion of foods to which you are sensitive. Eating foods that are inappropriate for your body creates inflammation that blocks absorption of nutrients necssary for creating energy. This blockage of absorption then deprives your body of the necessary building blocks for qi and blood. If you are finding that the above recommended diet and lifestyle techniques are not having much impact, consider getting yourself tested for potential dietary culprits.

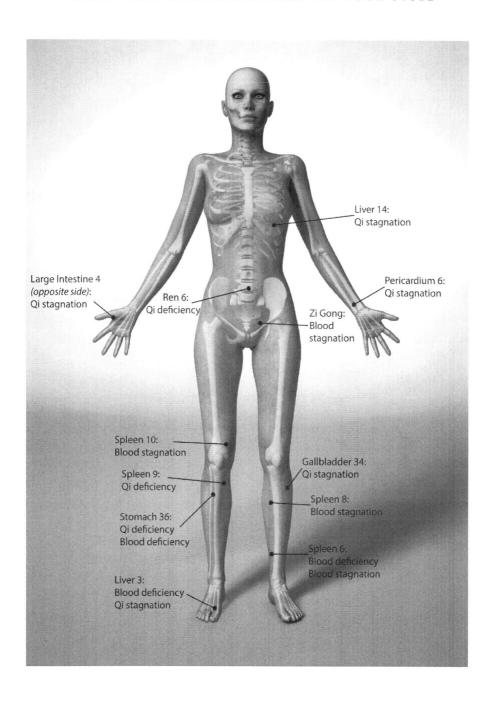

Liver 14:
Qi stagnation

Large Intestine 4
(opposite side):
Qi stagnation

Ren 6:
Qi deficiency

Pericardium 6:
Qi stagnation

Zi Gong:
Blood
stagnation

Spleen 10:
Blood stagnation

Spleen 9:
Qi deficiency

Gallbladder 34:
Qi stagnation

Spleen 8:
Blood stagnation

Stomach 36:
Qi deficiency
Blood deficiency

Spleen 6:
Blood deficiency
Blood stagnation

Liver 3:
Blood deficiency
Qi stagnation

Blood Deficiency

The goal when treating blood deficiency is to refrain from foods and exercises that "burn" our blood, while supplementing this life-supporting, nutritive substance. Often, blood-deficient people do not have many symptoms of difficult menstruation. However, if left unchecked, long-term blood deficiency can lead to difficulty conceiving.

Diet

Add:

- Meat is one of the best sources of the bio-identical nutrients our body requires when suffering from severe blood deficiency. Unfortunately, many vegetarians will have difficulty supplementing blood without adding meat to their diets, but the foods below will help tremendously.

- Vibrant-colored berries

- Dark, leafy, green vegetables

- Recommended foods for qi deficiency

Avoid:

- Excessively spicy foods

- Alcohol (no more than one glass of wine per night)

- Coffee (no more than eight ounces of coffee per day)

Exercise

The quintessential blood-deficient woman is a slender endurance-exercise machine. Although exercise is very important for our body, it can be easy to overdo it. Marathon running and other strenuous endurance sports deplete our blood by forcing our bodies to use precious resources to repair the damage created through exercise. Additionally, our bodies were designed to see excessive exercise as a sign of stress, putting extraneous body tasks such as menstruation and fertility on the back burner as a nonessential body function. If you are suffering from blood deficiency and fit this description, it is essential that you tone down excessive exercise and choose to rest more—especially during menstruation.

Other self-care

Acupressure (see instructions under Qi Deficiency)—Stomach 36, Spleen 6, Liver 3

Food sensitivity testing (see explanation under Qi Deficiency)

Qi Stagnation

The treatment of qi stagnation requires the incorporation of foods and exercises that invigorate our body and improve the circulation of energy, as well as strategies to manage emotional stress.

Diet

When suffering from qi stagnation, it is important to eat relatively small and regular meals. Eating large meals of foods that are difficult to digest can compound stagnation, while small, regular meals encourage free flow and easy digestion. There aren't necessarily specific foods to add or avoid if you are suffering from qi stagnation. However, it is recommended that you follow the healthy food guidelines outlined under qi and blood deficiency.

Exercise

Exercise is paramount if you suffer from qi stagnation. Cardio exercises are particularly effective at moving qi to prevent difficult PMS (including moodiness, bloating, and breast tenderness), while encouraging regular and pain-free menstrual cycles.

Other self-care

Mindfulness meditation—stress management is key for treating qi stagnation. In fact, emotional stress is often the sole *cause* of qi stagnation. Stress causes our muscles and our blood vessels to contract, creating a fight-or-flight reaction in the body called a sympathetic response. Over time, this interrupts flow of everything in our body—including our menstrual flow—and increases the emotional distress we feel during PMS. Cultivating a mindfulness practice and seeking emotional support is one of the most effective self-care strategies for qi stagnation.

Acupressure (see instructions under Qi Deficiency)—Liver 3, Large Intestine 4, Gall Bladder 34, Liver 14, Pericardium 6

Blood Stagnation

Blood stagnation can either be caused by old trauma such as a surgery, injury, or a difficult birth, or long-standing qi stagnation. When treating blood stagnation, it is important to improve circulation in the body while assisting in detoxification, since long-standing stagnation interrupts metabolism and elimination. Blood stagnation is considered a more serious condition because Blood stagnation is most related to gynecological diseases including endometriosis, uterine fibroids, and polycystic ovarian syndrome (PCOS). Although self-care is very helpful when managing blood stagnation, seeking expert care is necessary to receive full benefit from holistic care.

Diet

Using diet to treat blood stagnation, follow instructions from all of the above listed imbalances. Additionally, it will be important to choose foods that are detoxifying to the body, while improving efficient elimination.

Add:

- Detoxifying vegetables such as dark, leafy greens

- High-fiber seeds and grains such as quinoa and chia seeds

Avoid:

- Excessive meat consumption (no more than five meals per week if blood stagnation is severe)

- Greasy and fried foods

Exercise

Similar to qi stagnation, when suffering from blood stagnation, it is extremely important to exercise. Cardio exercises improve circulation and naturally assist in detoxification.

Other self-care

Chronic blood stagnation is very difficult to resolve on your own. However, customized Chinese herbs are exceptional at dredging up old stagnation. Part of your self-care if you are suffering from severe blood stagnation will be choosing to make your healing a priority by seeing a specialist.

Abdominal massage is one of the few truly healing techniques you can perform on your own for blood stagnation because it focuses the treatment on your reproductive organs. However, refrain from deep abdominal massage if you have an IUD, flared cysts, or fibroids. See the chapter on uterine alignment for more information.

Acupressure (see instructions under Qi Deficiency): Spleen 6, Spleen 8, Spleen 10, Zi Gong Xue

Avoid tampons and try menstrual cups and reusable pads. This is especially important if you are suffering from endometriosis, since tampons can prevent complete expulsion of blood, increasing the backup of blood in the uterus.

Reusable Menstrual Options

Menstrual Cups

These flexible, bell-shaped devices are worn internally, like tampons, but collect your menstrual flow rather than absorbing it. Menstrual cups can be worn up to 12 hours at a time, including during sleep or exercise. Most menstrual cups are made of healthcare-grade silicone and are reusable for years.

Cloth Pads

Cloth pads are a comfortable alternative that contain none of the plastics, adhesives, fragrances, or chemical gels commonly found in their disposable counterparts. They are machine washable and may be soaked prior to washing to prevent staining if desired.

Learn more about reusable menstrual options at www.gladrags.com.

The Next Step

Self-care is absolutely essential for achieving any lasting health benefits. The choices you make every day have a direct impact on bringing your body closer to optimal health and vitality—or further out of balance. As a society, we are led to believe that there is a pill that can fix everything, but in truth, we often have the power to heal ourselves. Your body is not lacking pills; it is lacking only the commitment it takes to love and nurture yourself. By following the guidance outlined above, you are choosing to say yes to yourself and your body. You are choosing to fight for the ability to feel connected to your body and the rhythms of nature through your menstrual cycle.

If you are searching for even greater healing, acupuncture and Chinese herbal medicine are exceptional catalysts for change, and are especially powerful medicines for true healing of our reproductive system. If your body has been out of alignment for a long time, or if you have experienced extreme trauma, you might require care above and beyond daily diet and lifestyle choices. If you are suffering from more serious conditions, such as infertility, difficult pregnancy or menopause, PCOS, endometriosis, or painful and irregular menses that remain unchanging, make the choice to put yourself forward and seek the professional support that you, your menstrual cycle, and your body deserve.

Reflection Prompts

As you reflect on this chapter, consider your relationship with your menstrual cycle. Is it an inconvenience, a way to connect with your natural rhythms, or both? Note how your perspective toward your cycle impacts your self-care routine.

Do you feel balance in your life between work and play, rest and activity, your relationship with yourself and your relationships with others? How can you support yourself in seeking more balance?

Do you move your body? List five ways you can incorporate joyful exercise into your life.

Write down and reflect on any strong reactions that came up during this chapter.

Your Next Steps Toward a Better Cycle

- Pay attention to the signs that your menstrual cycle is sharing with you. Painful and irregular menstrual cycles are signals that your body is out of alignment with ideal health, and is an opportunity to make choices that support your highest well-being.

- Take the quiz to determine your TCM imbalance(s).

- Commit to changing at least one part of your diet, according to your TCM diagnosis, in the next thirty days.

- Choose to release one old habit that is no longer serving you in order to make room for a new, health-promoting activity—such as self-massage or exercise—according to your diagnosis.

- Practice acupressure daily for at least two minutes. Pairing it with a meditation exercise offers the added benefit of mindful relaxation.

- If discomfort or menstrual irregularity persists, seek additional support from a licensed TCM practitioner. You are worth it!

Beet, Fennel, and Avocado Salad

by Nicole Jardim

The 'b' in beets stands for B vitamins, especially folate—which is crucial to female hormonal health. Both beets and beet greens are rich in iron, a natural blood-builder and anemia fighter! Fennel is a diuretic and avocados are one of the best sources of healthy fat.

3 beets with the greens attached

1 cup fennel bulb, diced (save some fronds for garnish)

1 avocado, cut into one-inch cubes

1 small onion, coarsely chopped

2 oranges, zested and juiced

1 cup balsamic vinegar

1 T coconut oil

Remove greens from beets and set aside. Place beets in a pot and cover with one inch of water. Boil for twenty to thirty minutes, until a fork pierces easily through the middle of each beet. Drain beets and cool by running under cold water. Peel off the skin; it should come right off. Chop the beets coarsely.

Finely chop the beet greens and lightly sauté them in coconut oil. Mix all ingredients (except the avocado) and let sit for two hours. Add avocado and garnish with fronds.

CHAPTER 6

Detoxification for Less PMS

by Dr. Emily Lipinski and Gabriela Delano-Stephens

Did you know that before the average woman leaves her house every morning she has already been exposed to 126 different chemicals? This exposure is just from the creams, shampoos, makeup, and toothpaste she uses. Once she leaves her home, she is exposed to another slew of chemicals: the pollutants in the air, treated water, pesticides, hormones and fertilizers in food, heavy metals from food and dental amalgams, household chemicals, prescription drugs, and many other sources. We breathe them in, absorb them through our skin, eat them, and drink them. This bombardment of chemicals on a daily basis increases the toxic load in our cells and organs, which has been linked to a number of health problems including premenstrual syndrome (PMS). Detoxing your body on a regular basis reduces the toxin levels in your body, giving your organs a chance to catch up on their work—such as keeping your hormones in balance—which leads to healthier menstrual cycles and less PMS.

We all experience different PMS symptoms that can be attributed to various hormone imbalances, namely increased estrogen levels and decreased progesterone at different points in our cycles. Hormone imbalances can occur due to a number of different factors, such as poor diet, lack of exercise, constipation, stress, and excessive use of chemical-laden cosmetics. Dietary factors include an excess of refined sugar or carbohydrates, caffeine, hormones in meat and dairy products, and consumption of too much alcohol. Environmental factors include exposure to the estrogen-like substances in plastics, pesticides, and pollution.

When our detoxification pathways are not clear, we can build up an excess amount of xenoestrogens (substances that act like estrogens) and other various chemicals in our bodies. Ultimately, unhealthy lifestyle choices and diet, pollution, cigarettes, and exposure to chemicals can slow the process of how our body effectively processes and metabolizes various chemicals and hormones. In turn, chemicals that either act like hormones or play with the hormonal milieu in the body can build up, causing various adverse effects, including PMS symptoms.

How our bodies become toxic

The world we live in now has a lot more toxins than when our grandparents were our age, and unfortunately it is our own fault. In the last seventy-five years, a hundred thousand *known* chemicals have been developed, and we are likely exposed to a significant number of them. Toxic exposure isn't only from what we put in our mouths; it is also the detergents we use to wash our clothes, the perfumes we use to make us smell delicious, the creams we use on our skin, and even the bottles we drink from. Pollution is no longer just about the very visible, ugly smokestacks that are polluting our environment; it also includes many toxic substances that we cannot see or smell. And although you may not realize it, the pollutants in our waterways, in the air, and on land all over the planet affect our health. The health of our bodies is affected by the health of our planet.

As you can see by now, we are constantly exposed to toxins no matter what we do. This may feel overwhelming, but please don't fret! After you have read this chapter, you will have greater knowledge to avoid overexposure to toxins and daily habits to allow your body to detoxify more efficiently.

How our bodies detox

Our genetics may be an indicator of how we respond to toxic stress and our ability to effectively remove waste and chemicals from our body. An excellent way to increase detoxification is to help your body through nutritional and lifestyle modifications, which can be incorporated into your daily life to encourage your body to detoxify more efficiently.

Our liver is the primary way our body breaks down, repackages, and removes toxins from our body. This is due to a specific class of enzymes, known as the cytochrome P450 superfamily (CYP450), which are primarily located in the liver and are involved in metabolizing drugs, steroid hormones, and other toxic chemicals. To a lesser extent, the small intestine, lungs, brain, and kidneys also contribute to detoxification.

The liver performs two phases of detoxification:

- In **phase one**, the liver uses oxygen and the CYP450 enzymes to carry out a series of reactions, the most common being oxygenation, a process that helps to break down the toxins. This makes the toxins more water-soluble so they can be excreted in the urine via the kidneys. However, many products of phase one are not eliminated rapidly and must undergo phase-two detoxification to be eliminated from the body.

- **Phase two** involves taking the products from phase-one detox and carrying out various processes—predominantly a reaction called conjugation, which ensures the rest of the toxins are removed from the body.

When you decide to embark on your detox adventure, it is important that both detox phases are tackled by supplementing herbs and vitamins and implementing lifestyle changes such as sweating, dry brushing, choosing organic foods, and other daily habits you will learn in this chapter. If the original toxins are not properly processed, they can become more toxic due to chemical reactions within the body, making some of these substances more volatile or reducing the efficacy in which the chemicals are cleared in phase one. To make sure that both detox phases are addressed, you can supplement with specific vitamins to help with the process.

- **Phase-one activators**: vitamin B2, vitamin B3, vitamin C, magnesium, indole-3-carbonol, and iron

- **Phase-two activators:** n-acetyl cysteine, MSM, methionine, glutamine, indole-3-carbonal, onions, garlic, and protein

These phase-one and phase-two activators can be taken in the form of supplements or by eating foods that contain a high amount of these substances during your detox.

How can you detox?

Doing a detox for ten days or longer may seem daunting, but trust me: you will feel amazing afterward! It is important to note that there are many different ways to detox. Removing specific foods from your diet such as dairy, alcohol, gluten, refined carbohydrates, and sugars is a simple yet effective way to start clearing the detoxification pathways. Smoking must also be avoided during any type of cleanse. The longer you carry out such a diet the better; even two to three weeks can have very beneficial effects. Some people prefer an intense weekend-long juice cleanse, which is a great way to kick-start your body into healthier ways. Depending on your toxin levels, you may experience several side effects of your body cleansing out the toxins. These side effects can include fatigue, nausea, moodiness, headaches, irritability, or changes in bowel habits. To diminish such symptoms, it is recommended you prepare for your detox by slowly cutting out caffeine, sugar, and any other toxins you consume on a regular basis. Determine which kind of detox would work best for your lifestyle and intentions and stick to it!

Daily habits to improve your daily detoxification process

Enough of the technical stuff, let's look at what you can do daily to help your body detoxify more efficiently.

Water—Water is an essential part of the detox process as it is used by all organs and cells in our body. According to the Environmental Working Group (EWG), if you live an urban lifestyle, it is likely that your tap water contains trace amounts of chemicals and pharmaceutical drugs. All of our water systems are connected, and—no matter how treated the water is that goes through the sewers—trace amounts of chemicals can show up in our drinking water. Gross, I know, but the hard truth. Bottled water may also contain bisphenol A (BPA) if packaged in plastic. It is best to drink filtered water from your own filtration system or from bottled water that you know is free from plastics.

Lemon water—Drink a glass of warm water with the juice of half a freshly squeezed lemon every morning before breakfast to help your liver with its daily detoxifying duties. This will stimulate digestion and get your detoxification pathways working. If you have a citrus allergy, use one tablespoon of apple cider vinegar in water instead of lemon.

Shut-eye—Sleep seven to eight hours *every single night*. No ifs, ands, or buts. Sleep is an essential part of the cleansing process. It helps repair your muscle cells and rejuvenates your body. If you are lacking in the sleep department, you are more likely to have junk food cravings and less desire to exercise. Get better rest by avoiding caffeine, turning off your TV, laptop, or other devices before bed, and sleeping in a quiet, cool, and dark room.

Destressing—Make it to a yoga class, close your eyes and take three deep breaths in the middle of the day, slow down and smell the flowers, or take a different route on your way home from work. Little changes make a huge difference in stress levels. When you are constantly stressed, your body has a more difficult time with the many biochemical reactions necessary for effective detox and optimal health.

Exercise/sweating—Your skin is an organ, just like your liver, kidneys, or gallbladder. In fact, your skin is the biggest organ in your body!

If you look closely at your skin, you will see little pores, which are used by the body to breathe and to release toxins through sweat. This function is why it is so important to sweat on a daily basis, even when you aren't detoxing. When on a detox, it is best to avoid heavy exercise and focus instead on nourishing movements such as walking, yoga, or qigong to get your blood moving and your sweat glands activated, which helps the detox process. Other ways to encourage sweating are saunas or steam rooms. These methods increase the excretion of fat-soluble xenobiotics (synthetic hormones and certain pharmaceuticals that are lodged in your fat cells) and heavy metals.

Dirty dozen—Avoid pesticide-laden foods as much as possible. While we understand it can be expensive to buy everything organic, you can choose to purchase the most contaminated foods (the Dirty Dozen™) organic as often as possible, and the least contaminated foods (the Clean Fifteen™) not organic. Find a current list of the Dirty Dozen™ and Clean Fifteen™ at http://www.ewg.org/foodnews

Dry brushing—Dry brushing is a great way to open up your pores, remove dead skin cells, and stimulate your lymphatic system. The lymphatic system recycles plasma fluid known as lymph, which is comparable to blood plasma but may differ slightly. The lymph absorbs and transports fatty acids from the digestive system, and transports white blood cells to and from the lymph nodes and bones while helping to remove toxins from our body. Pretty impressive for a system that doesn't even have a pump! By stimulating your lymphatic system through dry brushing, you can increase circulation, improve your immune system, and reduce the toxic load in your body.

- How to dry brush: Use a dry natural-bristle brush (you can find these at a health food store or drugstore) and gently brush it over your skin, beginning at the extremities and brushing up toward your heart. It is best to dry brush before showering, as it is easier to loosen the dead skin cells on dry skin

Water therapy—Taking hot/cold showers is only one of the many forms of hydrotherapy, or the application of water to promote healing. Hydrotherapy is one of the oldest known therapies, used by many different cultures including the Egyptians, Assyrians, Persians, Greeks, Hebrews, Hindus, and Chinese to increase blood flow and improve circulation throughout the body. In turn this may also assist in lymphatic drainage, and can be greatly beneficial to incorporate into your detox regime.

- How to hot/cold shower: Just before you finish your shower, turn the water to cold (as cold as you can tolerate) for thirty seconds, and then back to warm for one minute. Repeat this three times, but finish the shower on cold. Try doing this as much as possible during your detox and attempt to make the thirty-second cold segments cooler each time for greater benefit. Caution: If you have any heart condition or arrhythmia, talk to your doctor before trying hot/cold showers.

Improve digestion—Improving your digestion can be as simple as learning how to chew properly. Make sure that you chew your food until it is a paste. It should take you at least twenty minutes to eat your meal. Avoid reading, computing, walking, or driving while you eat. By practicing mindful eating—or slowing down to enjoy your food—you give your body more time to realize it is full and experience a greater sense of satisfaction. Have you ever noticed how when you scarf down your food you feel like you want more right away? By taking time to truly enjoy your food by smelling, tasting, and looking, you allow for a more enjoyable and mindful meal experience.

Chia nightly—If you find that you aren't going to the bathroom as regularly as you would like (you should be going at least one or two times a day), then a good way to get your digestion moving is to put one tablespoon of chia seeds in a large glass of water and drink it before you go to bed. You don't have to soak the chia seeds. Make sure you are drinking enough water throughout the day because if you are a little dehydrated, you could end up more bunged up than when you started. Chia can absorb up to nine times its weight in water!

Cosmetics to avoid—Detoxify your cosmetic bag and by download-ing a sustainable shopper's guide to ingredients to avoid at http://www. davidsuzuki.org/whatsinside.

Gratitude—Healing has as much to do with the mind as it does with the body. This is also true with detoxing. Although the physical component is very important, we must pay attention to our emotional well-being as well. One way to get more in touch with your emotions is by expressing your gratitude for what you have in your life. Express your gratitude on a daily basis by writing it down in a gratitude journal. By focusing on the good things in your life, you will crowd out negative thoughts, detoxing your emotional being. The mind is a powerful tool; studies have shown that positive thinking increases life satisfaction and may even have a benefit in helping treat depression and cancers.

Detoxifying super foods

Apples—It doesn't have to be exotic to be a super food! Apples are high in pectin, a soluble fiber that helps your body to eliminate heavy metals and food additives. The high levels of flavonoids found in apples increase bile production in the liver, improving the digestive process and reducing cholesterol levels—all essential for happy detoxification path-ways. The high alkalinity of apples is essential in restoring the body's pH levels. You know what they say: an apple a day keeps PMS at bay!

Beets—We love beets! Beets contain betaine, a substance that en-courages the liver to get rid of toxins, thus speeding up the detoxifica-tion process. They are also a great source of fiber, which promotes liver function, improves the detoxifying capacity of the liver, and encourages elimination through the colon.

Berries—High in vitamin C, which helps to protect the liver and im-prove its detoxification capabilities, berries are an excellent choice during a detox. The high bioflavonoid content makes your liver extremely happy. Not only will they help with the detoxification process, but berries supply tons of nourishment as they are super high in antioxidants. The seeds in many berries are also excellent cleaners for your colon. Try to buy organic as much as possible, as most of them are heavily sprayed.

Celery—A natural diuretic, this will get the juices flowing, aiding in the elimination process. Celery is high in phthalides, powerful phytonutrients that lower high blood pressure, relieve inflammation, and stimulate the production of the enzyme glutathione S-transferase, which helps the body to detoxify specific chemicals. To boot, its high silica content is great for your skin and hair!

Chia—Chia is an outstanding food that is extremely high in both soluble and insoluble fiber. This means that it pushes things along in your intestine, helping with the detox process, and also absorbs water so it can literally grab on to toxins in your system and take them out with the trash! It is the highest plant source of omega-3 fatty acids—those incredible fats that make you smarter, happier, and more beautiful! Chia seeds are also high in a number of minerals such as magnesium, calcium, and iron, which are not only nourishing, but also aid the detoxification process. Chia seeds are a complete source of protein, just like meat. You can put them in your smoothies, sprinkle them on your porridge or salads, or just drink them straight up in water.

Cruciferous veggies—These vegetables include broccoli, cauliflower, brussels sprouts, kale, and cabbage. They contain indole-3-carbinol, which is important for hormonal balance because it literally carries excess estrogen out of the body when you have a bowel movement. These vegetables stimulate the body's natural detoxifying properties. Some people have a hard time digesting these vegetables because of the inulin, which is a fiber. If this is the case for you, exposing them to heat either by sautéing or steaming will help break down the fiber. Kale is very high in chlorophyll, which—because of its similarity in chemical structure to heme (basically blood)—is an amazing blood detoxifier. It is also extremely high in antioxidants and very alkaline. So get your kale on!

Ginger—A well-known anti-inflammatory agent, which can reduce joint pain, ginger is great for the nausea and upset stomachs that may happen during a detox.

Goji berries—These are an essential part of any detox. Their rocket-high antioxidant activity protects your skin and cells, while the vitamin C helps your liver to detoxify alcohol and recreational drugs from your system.

Lemon—These sour suckers cleanse and strengthen the liver, making it a more efficient detoxifier. They also increase the liver's detoxifying enzymes, improving its efficiency. Lemons contain high levels of minerals used by the body to detoxify, including manganese, which has been shown to help detoxify the body of heavy metals, and potassium, an electrolyte that helps with the water balance necessary to flush out toxins. High in vitamin C, lemons stimulate the production of bile, which carries toxins out of the body, improves digestion, and enhances the overall detoxification process.

Onion family—Leeks, chives, garlic, and onions are all members of this pungent family. These are excellent detoxifiers for the body because the sulphur-containing amino acids are necessary for specific liver detoxification pathways. The onion family promotes glutathione production, a compound used by the liver for detoxification of the caffeine and acetaminophen found in many pharmaceuticals. If you find that raw onions or garlic are too strong on your stomach, try cooking them. This makes them easier to stomach for most.

Turmeric—Right now this is the most studied food for its cancer-fighting abilities. According to a study done on cancer patients, turmeric has been shown to literally reduce the size of tumor cells. Although more clinical studies are needed, recent studies also show turmeric to be a promising substance to increase overall health. Turmeric contains a phytonutrient called curcumin, which stimulates the production of bile and supports the liver's detoxifying enzymes. It encourages glutathione synthesis and promotes gastric, colon, and liver cell function.

White and green tea—The bioflavonoids in white and green tea boost the production of detoxifying enzymes capable of converting carcinogens into harmless chemicals in the human body. By choosing organic you will reduce the toxic load from pesticides. Loose leaf is always better than bagged teas, as you avoid the chemicals used to make the paper bags.

Now you have the tools to embark on your own personalized detox. Grab a friend and do it together, or get your whole family in on it. We recommend you choose a time of year when you won't have too many social engagements. If you do, make sure you are prepared and take some healthy options wherever you go!

Reflection Prompts

Embarking on a detox can bring up deep emotions as your body clears out its system. Journaling during your detox is a useful exercise to track your emotions and how they correspond to your diet. Make sure to take extra time for yourself to reflect on the messages your body is sending you.

What are you grateful for today? Make a practice of writing down a gratitude list daily or weekly.

Which super foods in this chapter appeal to you most? How can you incorporate them into your meal routine?

Write down and reflect on any strong reactions that came up during this chapter.

Your Next Steps Toward a Better Cycle

- **Timing**—Choose an amount of time to embark on your cleanse and make sure you don't have any trips or events that may sabotage your efforts.

- **Buddy up**—Find a friend to join you on this cleanse. Doing this with a friend will help you follow through.

- **Prepare**—We call this a pretox. The week before you embark on your cleanse, start to reduce the amount of toxins you consume— particularly coffee, alcohol, cigarettes, sugars, and any other toxins you consume regularly. Do your grocery shopping ahead of time, and make sure you are well stocked so you don't fall into temptation. Make sure you will have the time to rest during your cleanse as well. Don't fill up your evenings and weekends; you might just feel like vegging out on the couch and reading during your detox.

- **Go!**—Start your cleanse following the daily habits outlined above. Make a copy of the daily habits and post them where you will see them every day. Keep a list of foods to enjoy on your fridge or on your phone so you don't slip up.

- **End your cleanse with care**—Whatever you do, don't have a hamburger as soon as you finish your cleanse! Once you are done with your cleanse, you will feel very sensitive to foods, energies, and your surrounding environment, so we highly recommend that you honor this by slowly introducing foods back into your diet. The longer you take to reintroduce foods, the better. If you suspect a food sensitivity, this is a great opportunity to investigate if you actually are sensitive to specific foods by introducing them one by one and assessing how you feel. Keep a journal. Introduce one new, potentially sensitive food type per day (dairy, eggs, corn, wheat, seafood) and track the results.

Aggarwal, B.B., Kumar, A., Bharti, A.C. 2003. Anticancer potential of curcumin: pre-clinical and clinical studies. *Anticancer Res.* 23:363-398.

Colborn, T., Dumanoski, D., Myers, P. *Our stolen future-are we threatening our fertility, intelligence and survivial? A scientific detective story.* New York: Dutton, 1996.

Crinnion, W. 2007. Components of practical clinical detox programs-sauna as a therapeutic tool. *Altern Ther Health Med* (2):154-6.

EWG Public Affairs. Press Release: Updated Tap Water Databases And Drinking Water Quality Analysis. 9 December 2009. Web 3 September 2013.

Giltay, E.J., Zitman, F.G., Kromhout, D. March 2006. "Dispositional optimism and the risk of depressive symptoms during 15 years of follow-up: the Zutphen Elderly Study.". *J Affect Disord* **91** (1): 45–52.

Jung, J., Oh, Y., Oh, K., et al. 2007. Positive thinking and life satisfaction amongst Koreans. *Yonsei Med J* 48:371-378.

Kleywegt, S., Pileggi, V., Yang, P., Hao, C., et al. 2011. Pharmaceuticals, hormones and bisphenol A in untreated source and finished drinking water in Ontario, Canada-occurrence and treatment efficiceny. *Sci Total Environ* 409:1481-8.

Tanner, C. 1989. The role of environmental toxins in the etiology of Parkinson's disease. *Trends in Neuroscience* 12:49-54.

Tindle, H.A., Chang, Y.F., Kuller, L.H., Manson, J.E., Robinson, J.G., Rosal, M.C., Siegle, G.J., Matthews, K.A. 2009. Optimism cynical hostility, and incident coronary heart disease and mortality in the Women's Health Initiative. *Circulation* **120** (8): 656–662

Tuma, R. 2007. Environmental Chemicals, not just overeating-may cause obesity. *JNCI J Natl Cancer Instit* 99(11):835.

Turner, Natasha, N.D. *The Hormone Diet Recharged* Toronto: Random House Canada, 2011.

Morley, C. *Best Detox Practices*, 2011.

Oliver, G. and Detmar, M. 2002. The rediscovery of the lymphatic system: old and new insights into the development and biological function of the lysmphatic vasculature. *Gens and Dev* 16:773-783.

Pizzorno, J. and Murray, M. *The Textbook of Natural Medicine*: Third ed, vol 1. Missouri: Elsevier, 2006.

Schencking, M., Wilm, S., Redalli, M. 2013. A comparison of kneipp hydrotherapy with conventional physiotherapy in the treatment of osteoarthritis: a pilot trial. *J integr Med* 11:17-25.

Bengmark, et al. 2009. Plant-derived health: the effects of turmeric and curcumionids. Nutr Hosp. May-Jun;24(3):273-81.

Benzie, I.F.F., Wachtel-Galor, S., eds. Boca Raton (FL): CRC Press; 2011.)

Lovin' My Green Juice

by Nicole Jardim

Green juice is my favorite way to start the day because it is a great detoxifier! Kale is the queen of greens, celery is a diuretic and digestive aid, lemon is a liver cleanser, and ginger adds a nice kick to the whole juice. What's not to love?!

4 kale or Swiss chard leaves

½ cucumber

2 celery ribs

½ bunch of parsley

½ lemon, with skin on

½ granny smith apple

1-inch piece of ginger

Juice all ingredients in a juicer and serve immediately.

CHAPTER 7

....

Menstruation in Ayurveda

by Andrea Shuman and Michelle Magid

Many of us have spoken to our OB-GYN about our cramps, PMS, bloating, etc, only to be offered artificial hormones such as birth control pills, pain medication, or even psychiatric medication. In my formative years growing up as a woman, I was on high-level pain medications for cramps, birth control pills that made me gain weight and left me emotionally imbalanced, as well as finally being given the Depo-Provera shot to stop my period altogether! It took more than a year and a half to regain my cycle after I went off the hormone shot. This experience inspired in me the drive to find out what was at the root of my difficulty with menstruation, why I had suffered so much, and what could be done about it. This search led me to Ayurvedic medicine, the traditional medicine of India, practiced for more five thousand years.

Normal versus Common

In Eastern medicine, the menstrual cycle is looked at as being one of the clearest ways to assess the overall health of a woman. In order to truly see what is going on in our bodies, it is important to draw a distinction between "normal" and "common." According to Ayurveda, menstrual cramps are not normal. That's right. Cramps are a common plague, but they are still an imbalance. Let's back up and talk about what Ayurveda says about healthy menstruation. According to the ancient texts known as the Charaka Samhita, the menstrual cycle should be regular and between twenty-seven and thirty days long. The bleeding should be bright red and should wash easily out of fabrics without staining. There should be no pain. The cycle should last between three and seven days and should be continuous rather than stopping and starting. Wow. How few of us actually have periods like this? Were the ancient sages living in some sort of fantasy world, or is there something we are missing here?

Society's reflection of the moontime

Western society historically has had a very conflicted and problematic relationship with menstruation. Many of us grew up during a time where feminism meant being the same and doing the same as men. We saw tampon commercials where women rode horses in white pants while having their periods…carefree and smiling. Where is the balance here? Is there a middle ground between ignoring our cycles and medicating them away, and suffering debilitation around the symptoms we experience during this time? I would like to propose that the truly feminist approach to menstruation is one that is profemale and honors the open and heightened sensory time that the cycle brings. The moontime is completely normal, but it is uncommon in our society to see it honored and treated with respect. By understanding our intrinsic nature and tendencies, Ayurveda can help us find the place within ourselves where peace is found in our monthly connection to nature, and joy is rediscovered as we learn that our innate intuitive abilities are increased during this time. By bringing our bodies and minds into harmony with our nature, we can experience periods that are healthy, comfortable, and often profound. What follows is a simplified explanation of the theory of Ayurveda as well as some helpful tips and insights to improve your monthly experience. We advise that you seek the assistance of a trained Ayurveda professional if you are experiencing more than mild discomfort.

Ayurveda 101

Ayurveda (Ah-yoor-vay-da) is the comprehensive holistic system of healing from India and translates as "the science or knowledge of life."

Ayurveda has been practiced consistently for more than five thousand years and has one of the longest and oldest knowledge bases for medicine in the world. Based on the principles of elemental medicine, Ayurveda looks at the basic building blocks of the universe and all things in it as the basis for its science. The elements, according to Ayurveda, are: ether (space), air, fire, water, and earth. These elements are literal at times, though more often metaphorical and a way of understanding life from the macrocosm in, rather than from the tiny cellular structures and atoms out. These elements are understood to be in each person and each thing on the planet and in the universe. In each individual human, different amounts of each element are present, creating a unique constitutional makeup of each individual.

Doshas

The doshas are, simply put, a combination of more than one element creating distinct body/mind types. Each type has some basic characteristics and some predictable health conditions. No one is the same; everyone is unique depending on the amount each dosha manifests in them. We will start with some basic understandings of each dosha. The doshas are Vata, Pitta, and Kapha.

Air and ether come together to create Vata. Vatas tend to be colder, thinner, highly creative and enthusiastic, bubbly, nervous or anxious, and have drier skin. We tend to think of them like a buzzing bee, due to their tendency to "buzz" from one thing to the next and their light nature. Vata disorders are often drier and lighter in character, such as constipation (dry stools that have a hard time passing rather than thick obstructions), anxiety, and painful cramping during menstruation. Vatas may suffer from vaginal dryness. Vata is the most vulnerable and unstable of the doshas and is responsible for the most health imbalances.

Fire and water come together to create Pitta. Pittas tend to be warmer than others, medium or athletic build, more "fiery" in passions and personality. They are driven, focused, captivating, and can tend toward anger and irritability when imbalanced, and make good teacher and leaders when balanced. Pittas can be thought of as a bull or tiger due to their strong leader tendencies and dominant nature. Pitta-type disorders are warmer, such as burning indigestion, loose stools, herpes, bacterial vaginitis, and menstrual symptoms like PMS with anger, headaches, and skin breakouts. Pittas may also experience cramping that is milder and warmer than Vata type.

Water and earth unite to become Kapha. Kaphas tend toward larger frames and features, including larger eyes, hips, and breasts, thick lustrous hair, and some difficulty losing weight. Kaphas are slower in manner and less motivated to movement. They make good, nurturing friends and tend to be the "mamas" wherever they are. Kapha disorders are more thick and sluggish in nature, such as diabetes, slow digestion, sugar addictions, and obesity. Kaphas can be thought of as a swan due to their wide, strong bodies and graceful, slow movement. Kapha menstrual issues are often fibroid masses, uterine congestion and blocking, delayed menstruation and leucorrhea (white discharge) as well as yeast infections. Kapha is the strongest of the doshas and least susceptible to disease.

All that said, you probably don't fall neatly into any single category. Most people have a dominant dosha or dual dominant doshas. You are unique, and simply understanding your nature and characteristics— such as warm or cold, dry or moist, light or heavy—can help you to use Ayurveda to assist you in achieving healthy and balanced menstrual cycles. Ayurveda uses the principle of antidoting with opposites to create balance. So if you are cold and dry, the treatments, foods, and medicines will be warm and moist.

At first glance, this profound medicine may seem complicated and obscure, but the more we use observation of ourselves and our environment to assess where we are, the easier the remedies become. For instance, if you notice that it is cold outside and your cramps tend to become worse in the cold, the use of heat, applied externally on the womb, would be recommended, as well as warm foods. If you notice your PMS or headaches become worse in the summer, choosing cooling foods, staying out of the direct sun, and avoiding exercising in the heat of the day can be practiced preventively. In the following section, we will look at some basic diet and lifestyle choices you can implement right away to start fine-tuning your relationship to the elements and your nature.

Lifestyle and diet

Ayurveda suggests that during menses women avoid unnecessary activity and exposure to cold and wind—especially with wet hair, which aggravates the Vata dosha and leads to increased pain and discomfort. We suggest considering meditation as a part of your daily routine, but especially during the menstrual time. You may find that meditation greatly reduces your symptoms on its own, as well as allowing your body, mind, and spirit to clue you in to the deeper reasons for imbalance. Additionally, it is suggested that women eat a diet that is nourishing and easy to digest. Ayurveda recommends avoiding sex during the menses as well, allowing the downward flowing energy (Apana Vayu) to adequately move and not be disrupted. For this reason, tampons are discouraged, especially for women with cramping. Soft, organic, reusable, cloth menstrual pads are the best choice for catching moon blood and tracking its condition.

Becoming familiar with your flow

We prefer to use lighter-colored pads that allow for visual inspection of the blood, although if you are using fun-colored organic pads, you can look on the tissue after wiping. Notice if the blood is dark red, bright red, pink, brown, or streaked. Notice if there is mucus, clots, or an unpleasant smell. Darkness and clots indicate stagnation, or inertia, in the cycle—the uterus leaving old blood behind to coagulate. Brown blood can also indicate stagnation, but may indicate dryness of the uterus and poor digestion (Vata imbalance). Very light periods and pink bleeding may be an indication that you are not really having a period at all, but spotting that could be associated with ovulation, pregnancy, or nutritional deficiency. Excessive mucus shows excessive Kapha and sometimes indicates heightened yeast presence. Unpleasant smell or burning may indicate the presence of unfriendly bacteria (Pitta imbalance). Ideally, you will have bright-red blood that easily washes out of your cloth pads. This is another reason that soft, organic cloth is the ideal catch for the menses.

Foods to avoid

What should you eat, and what should you avoid? Traditional Indian medicine relies heavily on the understanding of the energetics of digestion. Some foods will stoke your digestive fire; some will cause it to roar out of control, burning up nutrients along the way. Yet others will put it out completely. Finding the right balance is essential to avoid toxic buildup in the system, which can lead to increased menstrual symptoms. Sorry, ladies, chocolate does not serve you during your menses and can increase cramping and breast tenderness. Ice cream is another common craving that will make menstrual symptoms worse; it increases cramping, gas, and headaches. Spicy, greasy, and fried foods should be avoided, as well as foods with heavy animal fats. Spicy foods will increase mental agitation, headaches, diarrhea, and abdominal discomfort. Lastly, Ayurveda suggests that raw foods be avoided due to their cold, rough nature and the difficulty of digesting them. With all of those foods to avoid, what is a girl to do?

Foods to balance your cycle

Well-cooked veggies, grains, and legumes prepared with warming spices are a good choice, such as the classic vegetarian Ayurvedic dish, kitchadi, which is a mixture of mung dahl, veggies, rice, and spices. If you are not vegetarian and crave animal foods, good meat choices include chicken—especially dark meat—or a bone stock of chicken or lamb. If you tend to bleed heavily and become very fatigued on your cycle, choose blood-building foods such as dark-red beets and cooked leafy greens like chard and kale. If you have a history of cramping and clotting, drinking two ounces of aloe juice (the organic inner filet rather than the whole leaf, as indicated on the bottle) two to three times per day the whole week before your menses will help the uterus to expel old blood and function more smoothly. Your foods should be easy to digest, warm, and well spiced rather than hot and spicy. Foods that have special properties to heal the womb and balance the cycle are sesame seeds and untoasted sesame oil (better for cooking with), toasted sesame oil (for flavor), ghee, saffron, poppy seeds, dates, and almonds.

Herbs for menses

If you are not a trained herbalist, it is usually most effective to consult with a professional Ayurvedic practitioner to assess your constitution and make a custom formula specific to you and your menstrual challenge. That said, there are some basic herbal supports that are safe to try at home.

A classic western herb for uterine tonification is red raspberry leaf. At the Ahara Rasa Ayurvedic Centre, we make a tea to support healthy menstruation that includes raspberry leaf, red clover, nettles, oat straw, and peppermint. This nourishing tonic helps blood circulation to the uterus, provides vitamins and minerals, and supports overall energy and stamina. To get the medicinal benefits, take a handful of this mixture in a quart of hot water, steep covered at least thirty minutes, and drink throughout the day. You may drink this tea throughout your whole cycle regularly as part of your balancing routine, or narrow it to the window just after ovulation.

Aloe juice, as mentioned before, has amazing benefits. Aloe tones the uterus, expels stale blood, heals inflamed tissues, and has been found in studies to increase absorption of nutrients from food and supplements by two hundred times! If you have a colder constitution, you can add a pinch of dried ginger or pippili (piper longum) to warm it up.

Yoga for moontime

This is certainly a debated topic among yogis and Ayurvedics alike. Purest Ayurvedic practitioners will say to avoid all asana (physical yoga poses) during the first three days of your flow, and many yogis will say that asana practice is fine as long as you avoid inversions. As a woman-focused Ayurvedic center, we fall somewhere in the middle.

If you have a practice that is based on sun salutations (Surya Namaskar), like many Hatha practices, we suggest switching to moon salutations (Chandra Namaskar) either right after your ovulation or the week before your menses is due. You may also practice slow moon salutations during your cycle.

Additional poses to add to your short, relaxing menstrual practice include bound angle pose (Baddha Konasana), cow's face pose (Gomukhasana), one-armed camel pose (Ecka Hasta Ustrasana), and wide-legged child's pose (Balasana). You may also try other poses that combine a grounded seat, mild twists, and hip openers. Avoid inverted poses, challenging balancing poses, poses that increase the heart rate, and fast flows. This practice should be quiet, meditative, and contemplative. We do not recommend going to class during your cycle unless the class is designed for moontime.

At the end of your practice, as an alternative to regular Sivasana, we suggest queen's pose, which is accomplished by using a toga bolster under your back, lengthwise, a folded blanket under your head, and a rolled blanket supporting under your knees. Knees should be bent with the soles of your feet together. Lie back and place one hand on your womb and one on your heart. You may use blocks under your elbows for arm support if you wish. Take a great deal of time in this pose, at least ten minutes. Breathe into your heart chakra and let your exhale take the heart-energy through the womb, nurturing and mothering yourself. Take time in meditation after you sit up. Stay inward.

Self care for menstrual difficulties

Castor-oil packs are best used for stagnant blood, signified by old or dark blood, staining, clots, delayed menses, pain, and bloating. This therapy is not appropriate for those with weakness, scanty red or pink bleeding, or if you may be pregnant. To perform, you will need enough wool flannel to cover your whole abdomen twice (real wool is best), a bottle of organic castor oil, some plastic wrap or other protective material to prevent the oil from staining your clothing, and a hot pack or hot water bottle.

Begin by lying on your back and massaging the uterus and ovaries right above your pubic bone with warm castor oil. Massage in toward your belly button from your pubic bone and hips. Use circular motions clockwise, stimulating digestion and unblocking flow. Thoroughly saturate the flannel with castor oil until it is full but not dripping. Plaster it over your uterus and lower belly, and wrap the plastic wrap around to secure it. Place your hot pack over your belly and rest. The recommended time for use is ninety minutes for one full month on all days except the days you are bleeding.

This may sound like a lot, but the benefits cannot be overstated. The first cycle after this treatment will tend to be more painful as you pass old clots and stale blood from your uterus. This can be the case for up to two cycles. After that, a considerable change will occur. Blood should become bright red, and often pain will completely disappear. To continue this treatment for your second cycle, you should treat one to two times per week, then two to three times per month for the next cycle. After that, you can practice this treatment occasionally or once per month.

Alternate-nostril breathing

One of the limbs of yoga, pranayama, is directed breathwork with techniques for purposes including cooling the body, building heat, raising the spiritual energy, and solving various health concerns. Alternate-nostril breathing (Anuloma Viloma) is the pranayam we can recommend to nearly everyone to improve hormone balance.

This pranayam causes you to switch rhythmically from the use of the right brain to the left brain, creating a balance in the hemispheres. Holding your right hand in front of you with the palm toward your face, bend down the index and middle finger, leaving the ring, pinky, and thumb extended. Cover your left nostril with your pinky and ring finger, exhaling all the air from your right nostril. At the end of the exhalation, hold your breath out briefly for a couple of beats, but not long enough to cause any discomfort. Inhale through the right nostril, and hold at the top of the breath before exhaling, for a couple of beats. Again, not to the point of discomfort, but just slightly longer than the natural pause. Release your pinky and ring fingers from the left side, covering the right nostril with your thumb, and exhale through the left nostril. Repeat the same process on this side, going back and forth to establish a regular rhythmic breathing pattern.

The key to this exercise is doing it long enough. The goal for time should be fifteen minutes. Before you balk at the amount of time, this is among the most potent and corrective of all the practices available to balance the hormones. You can start at seven minutes and work your way up. Try setting a sweet-sounding alarm on your phone and placing it outside of the room but within earshot. This will help you avoid distracting yourself and allow you to relax, knowing that when the time is up, you will know.

Other moontime advice

Be gentle with yourself. Use moontime to scale back on interaction with worldly things. Although it sounds crazy to the average American, we recommend scheduling downtime and (gasp!) even choosing not to work on the first two days of your bleeding to honor the inward and uniquely psychic time that women are gifted to experience. If you work for yourself, this is, of course, much easier. We have cancelled appointments with clients on heavy days and learned over time to mark our calendars and schedule more lightly during the expected blood time. Keep the talking to a minimum. Expending unnecessary energy through a lot of chatter depletes your energetic bank account, and silence is like a savings plan that will help you to be more vital throughout the rest of the month. Your cycle is a blessing, connecting you to nature, the tides, and the moon. You are an expression of life in its poetic form— monthly birthing, building, growing, dying, shedding, and starting all over again. Every month you affirm your connection to your goddess, Gaia, Creatrix nature and in your love of this process and your healing lays your power. Enjoy your discovery. Om Shanti.

Reflection Prompts

With this chapter, you near the end of this guide—but your journey is far from over! True health is a lifelong process of deepening your connection with your body and we encourage you to celebrate your amazing work so far in whatever way feels natural for you. As you journal, you may wish to reflect on the personal growth you have manifested since first beginning this guide.

Consider the distinction between "normal" and "common." Which category would your menstrual experience fall under?

Which doshas resonate with you most? Why?

Write down and reflect on any strong reactions that came up during this chapter.

Your Next Steps Toward a Better Cycle

- Determine your dosha types based on the descriptions in this chapter.

- For some simple recipes, check out *Ayurvedic Cooking for Westerners* by Amadea Morningstar, and www.joyfulbelly.com.

- For more information about castor-oil therapy, read *Balance your hormones, Balance your life*, by Dr. Claudia Welch.

- Plan time to rest during your next cycle and mark it on your calendar. Even a two-hour period of rest and reflection will honor your body's work at the beginning of your cycle.

- Practice alternate-nostril breathing.

- Choose at least one yoga pose from this chapter and incorporate it into your self-care routine.

- Practice gratitude for your amazing body!

Curry-Spiced, Roasted Root Veggies with Tahini Dressing

by Nicole Jardim

I love root vegetables because they are very grounding, both energetically and physically. These fiber-rich sweet vegetables, combined with the Indian spices and cinnamon, make for a dish that will help build and warm you up from the inside out!

Curry-Spiced, Roasted Root Veggies

5 cups of root veggies, chopped uniformly (any combination of beets, turnips, rutabaga, fennel, carrots, parsnips, sweet potatoes, butternut squash, etc.)

2 T of coconut oil

¼ cup finely chopped shallots

½ tsp sea salt

1 T curry powder

1 tsp turmeric

½ tsp ground cumin

¼ tsp ground cinnamon

¼ tsp ground red pepper

1 big handful of parsley, chopped

Preheat the oven to 350 degrees. Heat coconut oil in skillet. Add shallots to pan; cook six minutes or until tender, stirring occasionally. Stir in salt, curry powder, turmeric, cumin, cinnamon, and red pepper; cook one minute, stirring constantly. Add shallot mixture to veggies and toss to coat evenly. Spread out onto a baking sheet and bake for about thirty minutes or until slightly browned. Top with parsley. Serve as is or with tahini dressing (recipe below).

Tahini Dressing

½ cup tahini

½ cup cilantro or parsley

1 clove garlic, minced

1 T wheat-free tamari or Braggs aminos

1 lemon, juiced

¼ cup water

Whisk or blend all ingredients together. Add more water until desired consistency is reached.

AFTERWORD

By now, you have a vast array of tools at your disposal to deepen your connection with your body and celebrate your cycle. Refer to this guide and your journal often to keep yourself on track as you make powerful body and soul changes that will positively affect your health for years to come.

Should you need additional support at any time throughout your journey, please visit www.anewcyclebook.com to connect with the authors of this book and share your story.

Remember to practice patience and gratitude with yourself. Change may not come easily, but it is always worth the effort. You are more powerful than you think! Congratulations on completing this very first step; we wish you the best of luck as you continue integrating these practices into your daily life. Welcome to your new cycle.

ABOUT THE CONTRIBUTORS

Tracy Puhl

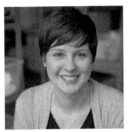

Tracy Puhl is the owner of GladRags and is passionate about helping women achieve period positivity while lowering their environmental impact. She is dedicated to serving her community and dreams of a world where all women are empowered to pursue their passion.

Inspired by the simple utility, earth friendliness, and comfort of cloth diapers, GladRags was founded in 1993 in Portland, Oregon. Today, GladRags is a small company with a big presence, promoting positive attitudes toward menstruation and making the environment a safer, cleaner place. GladRags can be found in health food stores and natural pharmacies nationwide. To learn more about how GladRags can help you create a happier, healthier period, please visit www.gladrags.com.

Aside from volunteering in her community and leading her growing business, Tracy enjoys traveling, reading, spending time with her family, and meeting new people. To contact Tracy, please visit www.tracypuhl.com.

Ashley Annis

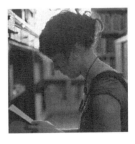

A modern-day Xochiquetzal (goddess of fertility, female sexual power, pregnancy, childbirth, and household crafts), Ashley uses her knowledge and passion to educate and empower women at all stages of life. Along with natural birth control classes and selling handmade menstrual pads, Ashley also aspires to work as a birth doula, lead feminine healing retreats and young women's circles, and become an expert on herbal medicine. To contact Ashley, please visit www.lovelyfertility.com.

Miriam Rosenberg, CNM

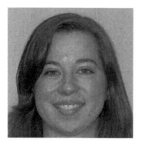

Miriam Rosenberg, CNM, is a certified nurse-midwife practicing in Portland, Oregon. She is passionate about providing respectful, evidence-based women's health care throughout the lifespan. She especially enjoys talking about birth control, women's sexuality, and vaginal health. She can usually be found catching babies, mushroom hunting, dancing like nobody's watching, and playing with her dog.

Barbara Loomis, LMT, RES

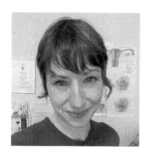

Barbara Loomis is a Restorative Exercise™ specialist and certified practitioner and educator of the Arvigo Techniques of Maya Abdominal Therapy˚ as well as a Chi Nei Tsang and Visceral Manipulation™ practitioner. She combines abdominal therapies with Restorative Exercise™ for reproductive and digestive health. Want to bring a workshop to your area or find out more about Barbara's services? Visit her website at www.nurturance.net. Or find helpful reproductive and alignment information on her blog at www.alignmentmonkey.nurturance.net.

Dr. Emily Lipinski and Gabriela Delano-Stephens, www.periodmakeover.com

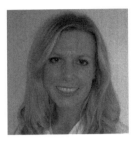

Dr. Emily Lipinski, ND, HBSc, and Gabriela Delano-Stephens, RHN, BSc, of www.period-makeover.com, are both food lovers and passionate about bringing the body back to health through natural remedies wherever possible. They started their website to bring awareness to women about the importance of attaining health through natural methods to balance hormones and reduce premenstrual symptoms.

Dr. Lipinski graduated from the Canadian College of Naturopathic Medicine in Toronto, Ontario, and is a member of the Ontario Association of Naturopathic Doctors. She strongly believes in addressing the root cause of a medical issue and using natural therapies either alone or in conjunction with conventional western medicine. She has a passion for women's health, including premenstrual syndrome, menopause, and antiaging. She is committed to helping her patients feel great and look their best.

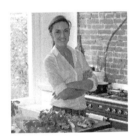

Gabriela is a holistic nutritionist and loves many aspects of food, from growing food and preparing meals to knowing how it works in the body to create optimum health. She works with clients from around the world, helping them to achieve their health goals. Gabriela is also passionate about yoga and is a certified yoga teacher. Yoga caught her attention with its power to calm the mind, heal the body, and release emotional tension as it taps into creative energy and allows us to transcend self-doubt.

Jessica Kolahi, LAC

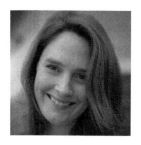

Jessica Kolahi is a hormonal health and fertility specialist, and the owner of Vitalize Acupuncture. In 2011, she received her Masters of Science from the American College of Traditional Chinese Medicine in San Francisco, and moved to Portland, Oregon, to actualize her vision of opening an integrative medicine clinic for women. With ten years of experience in alternative medicine, Jessica is passionate about educating women on how to heal themselves while cultivating awareness of the potential that all of us have to live a life of greater vitality and well-being. To contact Jessica, please visit www.vitalizeacupuncture.com.

Andrea Shuman and Michelle Magid, Ahara Rasa Ayurvedic Centre

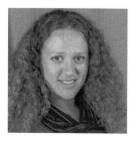

Andrea Shuman, Ayurvedic health practitioner and licensed massage therapist, has been in the field of holistic healing for more than sixteen years. Andrea is a graduate of the California College of Ayurveda and has traveled extensively practicing the healing arts. As a former sufferer of difficult menstruation and miscarriage, creating reproductive harmony became a mission for her personally and professionally. Through her own personal healing and study with inspiring women's health professionals such as Dr. Claudia Welch, Dr. Sarita Shrestha and Ysha Oakes, Andrea has made women's sexual and reproductive health and harmony a priority in her practice. As co-owner of Ahara Rasa Ayurvedic Centre in Portland, Oregon, and her own personal practice, known as Ayus Ayurveda and Massage, Andrea continues to love every minute of her work and feels honored by the presence of women who are ready to heal themselves.

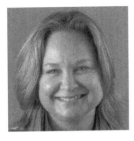

Michelle Magid, is co-owner of the Ahara Rasa Ayurvedic Centre and a skilled Ayurvedic practitioner. Michelle has a specialty in subtle yet profound healing therapies such as craniosacral therapy and crystal healing and practices the medical intuitive arts. Michelle left the corporate world behind to pursue her true calling in the healing arts and finds joy and fulfillment in facilitating authentic healing experience for women of all ages, especially those in transitions. Michelle has also studied with the aforementioned beautiful teachers as well as traveled extensively in India for study and life learning.

The skilled Ayurvedic practitioners at Ahara Rasa Ayurveda are available for in-person consultation as well as phone or video chat consultation for our clients around the country and the world. We are pleased to help guide you on your path to healthy menstruation.

To contact Andrea and Michelle, please visit www.ahararasa.com.

Emily Ruff

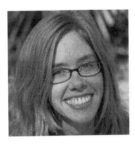

Emily Ruff is a community herbalist and director of the Florida School of Holistic Living in Orlando, which features a comprehensive curriculum, community clinic, and teaching garden. Emily studied herbalism across three continents under many indigenous healers, including herbalist Rosemary Gladstar, whom she credits as one of her biggest inspirations. Her academic studies include ethnobotany and women's studies, and she is a flower essence practitioner. Her line of products, Orenda Herbal, have been prepared since 2004 with love and locally grown ingredients. Emily has taught frequently at national conferences and regional events, and is also the organizer of the annual Florida Herbal Conference. Emily stewards an herbal urban homestead in central Florida, where in daily practice of meditation and digging her fingers in the dirt, the plants continue to be her greatest teachers. A frequently published author and dynamic teacher, you can learn more about her work and projects at www.emilyruff.com.

Nicole Jardim

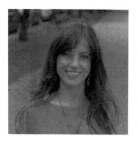

Nicole is a women's health coach and chief professional period fixer-upper at The Healthy Elements, the business she founded in 2010 to help women reclaim their hormonal health and feminine vitality naturally. She is the creator of Fix Your Period, a series of programs that empower women to heal their menstrual conditions in a fun and sassy way. She studied at the Institute for Integrative Nutrition and continued her training with Dr. Sara Gottfried and Jessica Drummond, two renowned hormonal health experts. Nicole passionately believes that all women should be active participants in their reproductive health, and she is dedicated to spreading this message. Nicole also cohosts a radio show called The Period Party, and you can find her on Facebook and Twitter. To contact Nicole, please visit www.thehealthyelements.com.

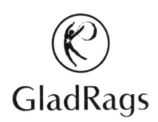

www.gladrags.com
hello@gladrags.com

Made in the USA
San Bernardino, CA
21 January 2015